Music and the Experience of Memory Loss

This book is a creative and critical exploration of the memory loss experience. Drawing on in-depth case studies based on primary research, interviews, approaches from music therapy, and theory from Derrida, Malabou, and Royle, it explores how we might better support people living with memory loss.

Telling the story of an interpretative phenomenological analysis investigation, this innovative book focuses on conversations with ten people living with memory loss in a nursing home, alongside interviews with the pioneering dementia campaigner Wendy Mitchell. The author argues that, for residents who are living with memory loss, both the nursing home environment and the memory loss experience are uncanny. She considers how archival impulses may manifest themselves at the end of life, before exploring theories of both artistic plasticity and neuroplasticity, proposing that the memory loss state might be thought of as a kind of neurodiversity. The book concludes with suggestions for future methods that alleviate disorientation for people living with memory loss and help with acceptance, the reduction of stress, and better outcomes across multiple disciplines and practices, including music therapy, community musicianship, and the nursing home environment itself.

A better understanding of how it feels to live with memory loss is necessary for the development and improvement of practices that are designed to help the memory loss community. This book is an invaluable contribution to research around memory loss, for scholars and practitioners interested in medical humanities, dementia, social care nursing, occupational therapy, and music therapy, among others.

Samantha Harrold is a writer, composer, musician, teacher, and medical humanities researcher. Her doctorate on the experience of memory loss is from the University of Sussex, UK.

Routledge Advances in the Medical Humanities

Medical Education, Politics and Social Justice
The Contradiction Cure
Alan Bleakley

Poetry in the Clinic
Towards a Lyrical Medicine
Alan Bleakley and Shane Neilson

Critical Humanities and Ageing
Forging Interdisciplinary Dialogues
Edited by Marlene Goldman, Kate de Medeiros and Thomas Cole

Palliative Care Nursing as Mindfulness
Embodying a Relational Ethic through Strong Emotion, Uncertainty and Death
Lacie White

From Loneliness to Solitude in Person-centred Health Care
Stephen Buetow

Ageism and Person-Centred Care
Rehabilitating Bias for Age-Friendly Practice
Stephen Buetow

Metacognition, Metahumanities, and Medical Education
Thinking Without the Box
Alan Bleakley, Quentin Eichbaum and Rachel Ellaway

Reproduction and the Maternal Body in Literature and Culture
Bodies of Knowledge, 1726-1818
Jennifer S. Henke

For more information about this series visit: www.routledge.com/Routledge-Advances-in-the-Medical-Humanities/book-series/RAMH

Music and the Experience of Memory Loss

Understanding Dementia as a Form of Neurodiversity

Samantha Harrold

Routledge
Taylor & Francis Group
LONDON AND NEW YORK

First published 2026
by Routledge
4 Park Square, Milton Park, Abingdon, Oxon OX14 4RN

and by Routledge
605 Third Avenue, New York, NY 10158

Routledge is an imprint of the Taylor & Francis Group, an informa business

British Library Cataloguing-in-Publication Data
A catalogue record for this book is available from the British Library

ISBN: 9781041072652 (hbk)
ISBN: 9781041117988 (pbk)
ISBN: 9781003639657 (ebk)

DOI: 10.4324/9781003639657

Typeset in Times New Roman
by KnowledgeWorks Global Ltd.

Access the Support Material here: www.routledge.com/9781041072652

For my daughter, Ophelia

For my son, Edward

For my husband, Ashley

Contents

Acknowledgements

I must begin by thanking Professor Ed Hughes and Professor Peter Boxall, who have been enormously supportive throughout their joint supervision of this research. It has been a joy to work with such creative, open-minded, and talented academics and I am extremely grateful to them both.

Secondly, I extend my sincerest thanks to Professor Nicholas Royle, for allowing me to take his brilliant words to my piano. It was a pleasure to work with such a precious stimulus.

I interviewed dementia campaigner, Dr Wendy Mitchell twice during this process, and those interviews (together with her three books) have had a great impact on this research. The suggestions for adaptations to nursing home practices that appear in the conclusion to this book are dedicated to her, with love.

Dr Kerry Andrew (composer, writer, and musician) and Douglas Noble (Live Music Now) generously allowed me to interview them about the creative process behind *The Sky Begins to Change,* and Dr Ming Hung Hsu (The Cambridge Institute of Music Therapy Research) spoke to me about current music therapy practices. These conversations were incredibly insightful, and I am indebted to them for their time.

Heartfelt thanks to my sister, and fellow musician, Stephanie Gordon, who interpreted and recorded all four of the reflexively written pieces that appear in this book. I was amazed by her musical talent when she first picked up a violin at the age of five, and she continues to amaze me now.

Love and thanks, also, to my late grandfather, who inspired this work by showing me how beautiful and brilliant the memory loss brain is.

My final word of thanks goes to my wonderful children, Ophelia and Edward, and my kind and supportive husband, Ashley. Being one-quarter of my family is my greatest privilege, and the love that I feel for the three of them will be *the very last thing.*

Chapter 1

Introduction

This book is a creative and critical exploration of the memory loss experience, in which I postulate that the memory loss state might be thought of as an alternate way of being, rather than a catastrophic loss of the self. Using innovative creative practice (including four reflexively written musical compositions and passages of creative writing), I tell the story of a two-month-long interpretative phenomenological analysis (IPA) investigation, in which I worked in a nursing home with ten people who were living with memory loss. The primary aim of the research was to consider whether a creative and critical approach to an IPA investigation might offer an insight into the memory loss experience, and I do this through analysis and discussion of five case studies. To begin, and alongside interviews with pioneering dementia campaigner Wendy Mitchell and theory from Sigmund Freud and Nicholas Royle, I suggest that for residents who are living with memory loss, both the nursing home environment and the memory loss experience are uncanny, which compounds the sense of a loss of home. Next, I turn to Jacques Derrida to consider how the data that I have collected can be looked at in terms of archival impulses, with a particular focus on how this manifests itself at the end of one's life for people who are living with memory loss. Finally, I look to Catherine Malabou to question what this research might mean in terms of theories of both artistic plasticity and neuroplasticity, before proposing that the memory loss state might be thought of as a kind of neurodiversity. I conclude by making suggestions for the way in which the findings of this research might shape future methods that alleviate disorientation and help with acceptance, reducing stress and leading to better outcomes across multiple disciplines and practices, including music therapy, community musicianship, and the nursing home environment itself.

Personal experience

The desire to carry out this research is driven by personal experience. My grandfather was diagnosed with vascular dementia in the summer of 2017, and we spent a large amount of time together between his diagnosis and his death in February 2019. Following his diagnosis, I read many books, studies, journal entries, and articles. At the time, and as a musician, I was interested to read about the use of music

DOI: 10.4324/9781003639657-1

as therapy for people living with memory loss, and, as such, I arranged, organised, and performed at several concerts at my grandfather's care home. The impact of the music was evident – upon hearing familiar music (Christmas carols, in the first instance), many of the residents appeared to 'wake up' (just as in the famous case of 'Henry wakes up'), singing words that they had known for many years, and then for a short period afterwards, they appeared more lucid, more awake, and more 'themselves'.[1] However, I noticed that when the period of lucidity started to fade and the residents began to 'fall back to sleep', they seemed confused, disorientated, and upset.

The concerts at my grandfather's care home were integral to the development of this study. Whilst they confirmed to me that music has the power to resurface memories, what happened to the residents afterwards seemed to be extremely unpleasant. I was also concerned by the way in which using music to 'wake people up' seemed to support the narrative of a need to re-establish a pre-dementia identity. This was the same narrative that I was seeing as I researched products on the memory market as I looked for things that I could buy to 'help' my grandfather with his dementia. It seemed to me that the aim of these products (such as talking photo albums) was to trigger memories from the past to prevent the perceived loss of identity that comes with the memory loss state. As I continued to read about and research the different products that were available, I was also struck by the repetition of the language used to advertise them. The words, *preserve*, *rewind*, and *reclaim*, were used on repeat to market products and practices that were attempting to counteract what was presented as a catastrophic loss of the self, and there was little that seemed to place any value on the memory loss state. I began to reflect upon this focus of pushing people backwards towards a pre-memory loss identity, and following several episodes in which I had accidentally frightened my grandfather by talking about the past, I changed my perspective and began to think about the value of the memory loss brain in the present and future space.

This change of perspective, which happened in June of 2018, thawed all the fear I had about my grandfather losing his memory, and it allowed both of us to spend many contented hours together until his death in February of 2019. To put it simply, we adapted to one another; he with his memory loss brain, and me with my changed approach, and we met somewhere in the middle. This enabled me to appreciate my grandfather in (what was) his current memory loss state, and I also began to understand the importance of understanding the memory loss experience. I took the time to try to understand the way in which my grandfather's memory loss was having an impact on how he was feeling and then used that information to make small adaptations to the way in which we spent our time together. For example, during our conversations, I avoided talking about the past, and if we listened to music together, we did so in the calm space of his room, rather than in the busy communal lounge. I took books of very short stories and textbooks with short chapters for him to read, and I also stopped showing him old photographs. All these minor adaptations noticeably reduced stress and disorientation for my grandfather, which made him calmer, happier, and more communicative.

This study is, of course, inspired by my late grandfather, and everything written in this book comes from a place of hope and a desire to make a valuable contribution towards an understanding of the memory loss experience. This is because I believe that a better understanding of how it feels to live with memory loss is necessary for the development and improvement of practices that are designed to help the memory loss community. There are times in this book when the suggestions that I make may seem unpalatable or even disruptive. Please read them knowing that this work has been conducted with the aim of improving the lives of the memory loss community, and that the ethos throughout is that an identity changed by memory loss is different, not less.

Key terms

For the purposes of this study, when using the words 'living with memory loss', I am referring to people who *self-identify as having problems with their memory.* Whilst those people may also have received a clinical diagnosis such as Alzheimer's disease, vascular dementia, or memory problems induced by liver damage, the clinical diagnosis itself is not relevant to this study. Therefore, I use the words 'living with memory loss' throughout.

How I work and how to read this book

I compose reflexively alongside my writing, whether the writing is creative or critical, or both. This is a stim which helps me to process what I am writing and thinking about. The pieces of music (over which I have little to no control) are varied and by the time I reach the double bar line at the end (if there is one), they have served their purpose. As such, it is the process of writing these pieces that is of value to me. The four pieces that I have composed during this process give an insight into the development of my creative and critical thinking that has taken place during the course of this study and are thus part of the story of this book. The compositions are significantly language based and include the use of speech fragments, so they may be thought of as pieces of writing, as well as pieces of music. The recordings of the compositions have been recorded by a fellow musician, and the recordings, scores, and programme notes are available to access online, with signposts of how to do so placed at appropriate moments throughout the book. Please note that the recordings are interpretations of the scores, rather than definitive realisations, and are offered as examples of how the pieces might sound in performance.

This book is the story of an IPA investigation, as well as the research project itself. At times when the writing might be categorised as 'creative', please note that, whilst this may be the case, my intention is to convey real-world and lived experiences. The accounts that are offered, particularly at the point of analysis, are written with respect, care, honesty, and a strong awareness of the ethical responsibility that comes with writing about the lives and experiences of other people.

Creative and critical

I am a writer, composer, musician, and teacher. This research could not have been carried out without this body of expertise, and it is this that defines this project as that of a creative practitioner. As such, this is an integrated multi-media creative and critical writing book that gathers together work that spans critical analysis, essayistic creative non-fiction, poetry, memoir and life writing, interviews, engaged research, creative engagements with existing writing, and new musical compositions.

Research questions

The primary research question for this study is, "How can a creative and critical approach to an IPA investigation offer an insight into the memory loss experience?"

The secondary research question for this study is, "How can data gathered during a creative and critical IPA investigation inform suggestions for adaptations across a range of practices?"

Hypothesis

My hypothesis is that our current cultural perception of the value of the memory loss brain can be defined by what Anne Davis Basting calls, "self = memory" and "loss of memory = loss of self."[2] To put it simply, we do not value the memory loss state, and, once a person who is living with memory loss enters a phase in which they lose the ability to connect with their memories from the past (or so we think), we believe that they have lost their identity, and, therefore, their sense of self. This is evident in the way in which we think about and treat people who are living with memory loss and can be seen across multiple disciplines and practices. These include, but are not limited to, artistic representations, neuronovels, therapy designs, and nursing home protocols. For example, a music therapy session is considered to be successful if music triggers a period of lucidity for a person who is living with memory loss, meaning that the person is able to access memories from the past, and nursing homes play 'nostalgic' music and are filled with objects from residents' pasts to trigger memories and remind residents of the home that they have left behind. The problem with these practices is, whilst they are well-meaning, they (a) take place without an understanding of the negative impact that they can have upon the memory loss experience and (b) support Davis Basting's "self = memory" and "loss of memory = loss of self,"[3] which makes it impossible for a memory loss brain to hold value in the present and future space. Unfortunately, this leads to practices that are distressing and disorientating for the memory loss community. However, if policy makers had a better understanding of the memory loss experience, it would be possible to (a) adapt practices accordingly to alleviate disorientation and help with acceptance, reducing stress and leading to better outcomes across multiple disciplines and practices, and (b) ensure that practices were accessible, inclusive, and kind.

Methodology

The methodology chosen for this research project was IPA. IPA is a participant-led qualitative methodology in which the researcher must apply their creative and interpersonal skills to create tasks that allow the participant to share their lived experiences, which are then examined in detail by the researcher. The personal experiences of an IPA researcher feature heavily in the research data that is gathered, and I employed my skills as a writer, composer, musician, and teacher throughout the fieldwork. As such, and as is the nature of all IPA studies, I feature heavily in the resulting archive, and this study is non-replicable.

Main findings

The memory loss experience is uncanny. People who are living with memory loss live with a constant feeling of vague familiarity; it is a life of the vaguely familiar. When someone who is living with memory loss moves to a nursing home (which usually happens following a lengthy and unsettling stay in a hospital, and, therefore, a break from being in their own home), the attempts that are made to make the nursing home environment 'homely' (most commonly by filling the space with familiar objects and familiar music and sounds) can generate a further feeling of uncanniness, which, at best, can bring about extreme confusion, disorientation, and fear. At worst, it can render the nursing home environment unlivable.

It is helpful to think of the memory loss state as a kind of neurodiversity. People who are living with memory loss can become overwhelmed if they attempt to focus on more than one thing at a time. This is due to the sensory sensitivities that come with the neurodiverse nature of the memory loss state and can prompt people who are living with memory loss to 'switch off' or become disorientated or distressed.

The memory loss brain is an intelligent brain. People who are living with memory loss are able to plasticly adapt to their memory loss state, and the destructive nature of the memory loss state increases the memory loss brain's polymorphic ability. There is never a loss of self; people who are living with memory loss are capable of adapting and changing so that their identity may survive. This ability to adapt goes beyond the capability to protect what is already there and demonstrates an ability to learn *new* things. This is key to the ethos of this study for two reasons. Firstly, it is in direct contrast to the way in which we are conditioned to think about the memory loss experience. Secondly, it allows us to think about the memory loss state as something that holds value in the present and future space, thus opening the possibility for a shift in the way in which we think about and treat people who are living with memory loss.

Layout of book

In the following chapter, I begin to explore whether a better understanding of the memory loss experience might shift the current cultural perception of the value of the memory loss brain. I look at the way in which the negative language of the Sacksian neuronovel provoked a shift in feeling about the memory loss experience. I then look at representations of memory loss in the genres of film, theatre, and music, and the discussion is punctuated by two interludes. The first of these focuses upon a composition that uses speech fragments from people who are living with memory loss called *The Sky Begins to Change*, and the second focuses upon current music therapy models. I conclude by considering how the literary work of Dr Wendy Mitchell is beginning to disrupt the Sacksian narrative. The chapter concludes with an introduction to *Spin*: A conflict composed for the mouths and bodies of 4–400 performers, using speech fragments taken from the existing literature.

In Chapter 3, I begin to offer a new insight into the memory loss experience with the analysis and discussion of five case studies. In the first case study, the participant demonstrates that, whilst listening to music provokes a period of increased lucidity, this can have a negative impact. The participant in the second case study is a woman who, although previously a competent musician, struggled to listen to music as her memory loss progressed because her sense of hearing had changed. In the third case study, the participant reveals the time-travelling nature of the memory loss experience via her complicated relationship with memory and environmental sounds. In the fourth case study, I tell the story of a concert that took place in a dying woman's bedroom which 'woke her up' to the point where she was able to speak for the first time in many years. And in the final case study, the participant gives an example of the way in which the memory loss brain is able to manipulate the prosthetic to protect the truth. The chapter also includes introductions to two musical compositions and their recordings. The first of these is called *Strange World*: An environmental sound chance piece, composed in response to the unpleasant and over-stimulating sound world of the nursing home environment. The second is named *Sphere*: A chance piece written for the mouths, tongues, and fingertips of ten performers using speech fragments from study participants who were living with memory loss.

Chapter 4 begins with the suggestion that, for people who are living with memory loss, both the memory loss experience and the nursing home environment are uncanny. I then consider how the data that I have collected can be looked at in terms of archival impulses, with a particular focus on how this manifests itself at the end of one's life for people who are living with memory loss. I then question what this research might mean in terms of theories of both artistic plasticity and neuroplasticity, before proposing that the memory loss state might be thought of as a kind of neurodiversity. I conclude by postulating that the memory loss brain is an intelligent brain that borders on the magical.

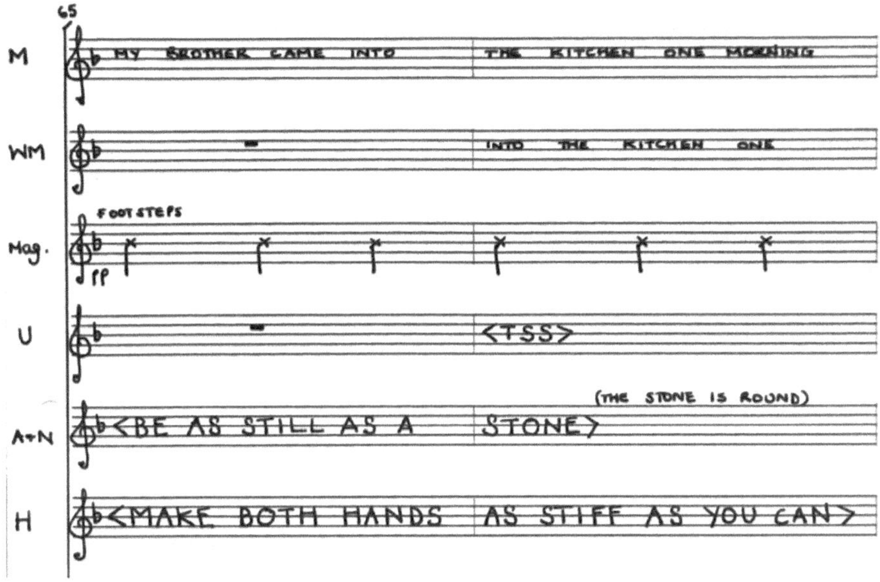

Figure 1.1 Excerpt from *Marbles*, taken from Appendix A. P1.

Please go to www.routledge.com/9781041072652 to listen to this and to read the score.

In Chapter 5, I postulate that a memory loss state can be thought of as an alternate way of being, and use the data collected to make suggestions for adjustments to the fields of music therapy, community musicianship, and the nursing home environment itself.

A note on *Marbles*

What follows this chapter is a musical score named *Marbles* (Figure 1.1), which was composed using speech fragments written by Nicholas Royle. Some of the fragments are taken from Royle's book, *Mother: A Memoir*, and others are taken from an interview with Royle in July of 2021.[4,5] In *Mother*, Royle offers a compelling and often mortifying account of his mother's Alzheimer's disease. Royle's words, I feel, capture something of where we are now, in our current cultural relationship with the memory loss experience. As such, I include my creative response to them here, as a starting point.

Notes

1 Music and Memory (2020) *Help spread the music* [Online] Available at: https://musicandmemory.org.uk/ [Accessed: October 19th, 2020]

2 Davis Basting, A. (2009) *Forget Memory.* Baltimore: The Johns Hopkins University Press, p. 24.

3 Davis Basting, A. (2009) P24.
4 Royle, N. (2020) *Mother: A Memoir.* Oxford: Myriad.
5 Appendix E. www.routledge.com/9781041072652

Bibliography

Davis Basting, A. (2009) *Forget Memory*. Baltimore: The Johns Hopkins University Press.

Music and Memory (2020) *Help spread the music* [Online] Available at: https://musicandmemory.org.uk/ [Accessed: October 19th, 2020]

Royle, N. (2020) *Mother: A Memoir*. Oxford: Myriad.

Chapter 2

Sacks, Mitchell, and the question of value

> "Self = memory" and "loss of memory = loss of self"[1]
>
> – *Anne Davis Basting, Forget Memory*

In this chapter, I will begin to explore whether a better understanding of the memory loss experience might shift the current perception of the value of the memory loss brain. I'll consider how the formula "self = memory" and "loss of memory = loss of self" became the current and often-deployed cultural narrative by looking at creative responses to the memory loss experience from the 1980s onwards.[2] I shall start by looking at titles of literary publications from the 1980s, before considering how the negative language used in the Sacksian neuronovel provoked a shift in feeling about the memory loss experience. I will look at representations of memory loss in the genres of film, theatre, and music, and the discussion will be punctuated by two interludes. The first of these will be interviews with composer and writer Dr Kerry Andrew and Douglas Noble from Live Music Now about a composition that uses speech fragments from people who are living with memory loss called *The Sky Begins to Change*, and the second will be an interview with Dr Ming Hung Hsu from the Cambridge Institute for Music Therapy Research about current music therapy models designed for people living with memory loss. I shall then look at the way in which the narrative arc is beginning to change, by considering how the literary work of Dr Wendy Mitchell is starting to disrupt the Sacksian narrative, before concluding by offering *Spin*; an experimental conflict for mouths and bodies that uses the polarising speech fragments from this literature to encourage a new approach to listening and seeing.

Although Alzheimer's took its name from Dr Alois Alzheimer in 1906, memory loss in elderly patients was largely attributed to mental illness or the natural ageing process until as recently as the 1970s, with the disease only being accepted by the American National Institute of Aging in 1978. In the years that followed, and despite a large amount of public interest and concern (A "Dear Abby" column about Alzheimer's received 30,000 responses in 1980), the early artistic response to the disease was surprisingly sparse.[3] Very early publications include books such as *The 36 Hour Day*, by Nancy Mace and Peter Rabins, and *The Myth of Senility: The*

DOI: 10.4324/9781003639657-2

Truth about the Brain and Aging, by Robin Marantz Henig, both of which were first published in 1981, and attempt to de-mystify the memory loss experience using a combination of practical advice and accessibly written neuroscience.[4] However, these initial texts were followed by several years of hiatus from the arts, with the development of the emerging cultural landscape being formed instead by the American government. In 1982, President Ronald Reagan declared that the fourth week in each November would become National Alzheimer's Disease Awareness Week, and the first public service announcement about Alzheimer's aired. In 1983, The House Select Committee on Aging held hearings on senility and stereotyping and The Senate Subcommittee on Aging held hearings on living with Alzheimer's.[5] By 1984, the cultural relationship with Alzheimer's had changed, as had the literary relationship with the disease, with a December edition of *Newsweek* printing, "The Agony of Alzheimer's Disease" on its cover, and publishing the article, "*A Slow Death of the Mind*" by Matt Clark, which was a far cry from the far gentler writing of Mace and Rabins and Marantz Henig of 1981.[6] Then, in 1985, Oliver Sacks' neuronovel, *The Man Who Mistook His Wife for a Hat,* was published.[7]

Oliver Sacks

Oliver Sacks was a physician, author, and professor of neurology. In his writing, Sacks persuades us that we must trust his ideas by framing his thoughts as the outcome of an ethnographic, reflexive, and qualitative research process. He takes the Freudian approach of positioning himself within the stories of his time spent with his patients (his presence is always at the forefront of the narrative) before socratically questioning a 'problem' that he has found in order to either confirm an existing theory about the brain or to develop a new one, or, as Jason Tougaw has it in, *The Elusive Brain*[8]:

> Sacks's case histories tend to follow a narrative pattern. A person experiences brain illness or injury that alters identity; Sacks's interactions with his suffering subjects raise perplexing questions about the brain, and these send him off on tours of the neurological literature; together, he and his subjects collaborate on a process of discovery that involves resurrecting insights lost in the history of neurology or creating new ones.[9]

Sacks uses this approach, in various forms, in all of his texts, and, although he is not the only writer in this genre, his work is extremely influential, and therefore, important to this study, because, as Tougaw writes, "Oliver Sacks may not have invented neuromania, but he was certainly the Western world's most influential neuromaniac – in literature as much as in other cultural spheres. He made a career of writing more prolifically about the brain and identity than any other writer of the twentieth century."[10]

The note on the back of my edition of *The Man Who Mistook His Wife for a Hat*, states, "In this most extraordinary book, Oliver Sacks recounts the stories of patients lost in the bizarre, apparently inescapable world of neurological disorders. These are case studies of people who have lost their memories and with them the greater part of their pasts."[11] This book, in which Sacks recounts stories of people that he has worked with during his neurological studies (most of whom are living with memory loss) is widely read (my cover claims, "The Million Copy Best-seller!"), and the way in which Sacks uses language in the text has had a noticeable impact on the way in which we think about memory loss.[12]

My critique of Sacks, and the suggestions that I make about his impact, are specific to his writing, and the way in which he communicates his ideas, particularly in *The Man Who Mistook His Wife for a Hat*, which, in this context, I am reading more as a piece of influential literature that has been consumed extensively within popular culture, than as science. Sacks was frustrated by the 'deficit' model of Western biomedicine, and he positions his work as extending the holistic neurology of Kurt Goldstein and romantic neurology of Aleksander Luria. However, his difficulty in articulating this in his writing means that that positionality is often lost, meaning that the text is read in a way that was, perhaps, unintended by the author. This is problematic for the work of Sacks and has led to a strong critique of his work in the field of disability studies, with Professor of Disability Research, Tom Shakespeare, famously referring to him as, "The man who mistook his patients for a literary career."[13]

'The Lost Mariner' is a chapter (or clinical tale) in *The Man Who Mistook His Wife for a Hat*, in which Sacks discusses the case of a man who is living with memory loss (what he calls a "peculiar, uncanny horror"), due to a diagnosis of Korsakoff's syndrome, who he describes as the, "charming, intelligent, memoryless Jimmie G."[14,15,16] The opening epigraph from Luis Buñuel reads, "You have to begin to lose your memory, if only in bits and pieces, to realise that memory is what makes our lives. Life without memory is our coherence, our reason, our feeling, even our action. Without it, we are nothing…(I can only wait for the final amnesia, the one that can erase an entire life, as it did my mother's)."[17] Opening the chapter in such a way suggests to the reader that the theme of the chapter will be that the loss of one's memory is catastrophic and is not a state that can be 'lived with'. However, Sacks attempts to challenge this idea as he turns his attention to trying to look beyond the memory loss of Jimmie G. He quotes advice from his mentor, Aleksander Luria as saying, "There is little or no hope of any recovery in his memory. But a man does not consist of memory alone. He has feeling, will, sensibilities, moral being – matters of which neuropsychology cannot speak."[18] Sacks acts on this advice by describing both the powerful relationship between Jimmie G. and his brother, and the profound impact that engagement with spirituality and music has upon his patient. He writes that Jimmie G. was, "so personable, so likable, so quick and intelligent" and makes genuine attempts to write about Jimmie G.'s memory loss state in a positive way.[19] The chapter ends with, "Perhaps there is a philosophical as well as clinical lesson here: that in Korsakov's, or dementia, or other such catastrophes, however great the organic brain damage and Humean dissolution, there remains the undiminished possibility of reintegration by art, by communion, by touching the human spirit: and this can be preserved in what seems at first a hopeless state of neurological devastation."[20] Whilst Sacks is attempting to offer a more positive view of the memory loss state, his use of language ("other such catastrophes") places the idea of the memory loss state in a negative space. He also makes use of "preservation" and "reintegration" as he offers the 'hopeful' suggestion that a person who is living with memory loss can be 'pushed back' into their pre-memory loss identity. This, coupled with the opening epigraph, undermines Sacks' attempts to discuss the case of Jimmie G. as a person who should be cared for, and instead suggests that he believes that there is no value to the memory loss state and that a pre-memory loss state must be returned to. This use of language resonates throughout the text and leaves the reader feeling as though Sacks believes that a memory loss state is a catastrophic loss of the self.

Throughout the rest of the text, when talking about memory loss, Sacks oscillates between disastrous language (*devastation, damage, dissolution, hopeless, catastrophic*) and language that suggests the need to 'push someone back' into their pre-memory loss identity (*remains, possibility of reintegration, preserving, pushing back*), all of which are persuasively repeated many times throughout the book. By the end of the text, whether it is Sacks' intention or not, one is left feeling that (a) memory loss is a tragic, terrible, catastrophic thing, and (b) the only way to fix what Sacks calls, "a hopeless state of neurological devastation," is to try to find a way to push the person back into their pre-memory loss identity.[21]

It is easy to see how this pessimistic, black-and-white approach to his writing (which Sacks acknowledges as a feature of the study of neurology) has an impact on the way in which Sacks writes so negatively about the experience of memory loss. He writes, "'Deficit', we have said, is neurology's favourite word – its only word, indeed, for any disturbance of function. Either the function (like a capacitor or fuse) is normal – or it is defective or faulty."[22] In other words, for Sacks (and neurology in general), a brain is either normal or faulty. Therefore, when a 'normal' brain changes due to a neurological disease such as dementia, in the eyes of neurology, it becomes faulty. In brutal shorthand, for Sacks, normal brain = good, and changed brain = bad. The use of the word deficit is important here (not least due to its relationship with not having enough money) because it suggests a failure, a shortcoming, and a lack of something that is absolutely necessary.

Later, Sacks goes on to say:

> To be ourselves we must *have* ourselves – possess, if need be re-possess, our life-stories. We must 'recollect' ourselves, recollect the inner drama, the narrative, of ourselves. A man *needs* such a narrative, a continuous inner narrative, to maintain his identity, his self.[23]

What Sacks is saying here, is that, in order to maintain one's identity, a person cannot live with memory loss. Instead, they must do whatever is necessary to reclaim themselves by finding a way to access their memories from the past. In other words, living with memory loss is not a possibility for Sacks. For him, those with a memory loss brain must find a way to access their memories from the past, or they must accept that they no longer have an identity.

Anne Davis Basting

In *Forget Memory*, Anne Davis Basting (an artist, teacher, writer, and director of the Center on Age and Community at the University of Wisconsin, Milwaukee) writes:

> The formulas "self = memory" and "loss of memory = loss of self," which inform so much of our thinking about people with dementia and determine how we care for them, seem terribly simplistic once we recognise the intense complexity of memory.[24,25]

Here, Davis Basting uses a strangely simplistic formula to summarise the cultural perception of the value of the memory loss state, and she notes that this idea is often echoed in artistic representations of the memory loss experience, in which stories of people who are living with memory loss frequently adopt a narrative similar to that of a Greek or Shakespearean tragedy.

The 'tragic' story of the person living with memory loss resonates throughout artistic representations of the memory loss experience. In nearly all representations, people living with memory loss are represented as white, middle-class, and intelligent and have had a 'respected' career, most often as a lecturer, writer, or teacher, or sometimes as a nurse or a doctor for the NHS. The lack of diversity in these representations, however uncomfortable, is of no surprise when one considers the 'othering' and excluding impact of the Sacksian narrative from which they came. The reason for this memory loss stereotype, however misleading, is that a white, middle-class, intelligent protagonist makes for a better tragic figure at the point at which they lose their value due to the loss of their memory. Davis Basting writes, "As in Greek and Shakespearian tragedy, in which a fall is more pronounced when taken from the height of kings, these stories most commonly involve people who stand out, people with extraordinary hearts and minds."[26] In other words, using the tragedy format as a starting point means that, just as in Greek and Shakespearian tragedies, we are titillated as an audience from the outset by the knowledge that the hero will fall (or die) by the end. Adopting this familiar narrative path means that representations of memory loss often depict the memory loss state to be symbolic of a kind of blindness, amounting to an inability to see or recognise truth, which leads to a death of the self. This not only appeals to a public who thrive on the sensationalising of a 'fall from grace' which is fetishised by the media, but, perhaps even suggests that, in this context, the loss of one's memory might be thought of as a 'fatal character flaw', over which the character might be expected to have a level of control. Because of this, Davis Basting notes that stories of people living with memory loss often share many similarities. She writes:

> there is a sharp contrast between who the person *was then*, and who the person *is now*. These stories climax in a moment when the two worlds (then and now) come together to reach some sort of harmony. This climax is commonly a moment of sudden lucidity – in which a woman suddenly recognizes her husband, or a father clearly expresses himself to his son – but can also be a moment of clarity for the caregiver about his or her perspective of the disease.[27]

The examples that follow this path are plenty and can be found not only in artistic representations of the memory loss experience but also in mainstream news media, with one notable example being the coverage of President Ronald Reagan's Alzheimer's disease.

President Ronald Reagan announced that he had Alzheimer's disease in an open letter to the American people on 5 November 1994. In it, he writes, "I have recently been told that I am one of the millions of Americans who will be afflicted with Alzheimer's Disease."[28] He closes by writing, "I now begin the journey that will lead me to the sunset of my life. I know that for America there will always be a bright dawn ahead."[29] The announcement triggered an outpouring of collective grief which is demonstrative of our preoccupation with memory on a cultural level. Davis Basting notes, "This story barely needed explanation. It was enough to say 'President Reagan' and 'Alzheimer's' in the same sentence to convey the magnitude of this tragic fall."[30] When Reagan died in 2004 at the age of 93, the media cemented his fallen hero status by bombarding the American public with yet more stories of the tragedy of his Alzheimer's diagnosis, with little mention of his achievements and the fine age that he had reached.

There are countless artistic examples too that follow a similar narrative. One early example came in 1987, when the film, *Do You Remember Love?* was aired on the television. The story follows the later years of an esteemed professor of poetry named Joan who has Alzheimer's Disease. At the beginning of the film, Joan is introduced as a white, middle-class (the class signifiers in the film include an extensive knowledge and *memory* of literature and classical music) woman who is highly intelligent and successful. We first learn that Joan is experiencing symptoms of Alzheimer's Disease when she struggles to find her way to her classroom. Shortly after this, she is told that she is being considered for an illustrious poetry award. We are to believe that if she were to win, it would be the highlight of an already successful career. As Davis Basting has it, "Right away, we know these two themes – her increasing confusion and her increasing professional recognition – are headed for collision."[31] And indeed they do. Predictably, this tragedy takes the turn that it must, and we watch Joan's world unravel. She receives the award, but when she takes to the stage to accept it at a ceremony which is attended by her contemporaries, she becomes confused and cannot find her words (what worse a fate for a poet?, we are led to think), and then her husband George has a moment of clarity before joining Joan on the stage and making a compelling speech to the audience about Joan's condition. Joan's memory loss means that she publicly loses her identity as a professor and poet in this one tragic moment at the end of the film. Other examples that follow a similar plotline (fall from great height, collision of past self and new self, moment of clarity and final fall) are, *Iris* (2001) and *The Notebook* (2004) and there are many more.

Strangely, the late noughties and early 2000s saw artistic representations that glamourised the memory loss experience. Using amnesia rather than a diagnosis such as dementia so as not to frighten a younger audience, there were a series of films made such as *The Matrix* (1999), *Momento* (2000), and *Eternal Sunshine for the Spotless Mind* (2004), all of which use captivating cinematic imagery to make memory loss look exciting. The memory loss experience was even presented as being cute, in the form of the little blue fish named Dory, in Disney's *Finding Nemo* (2003). However, what is unusual about Dory is that her memory loss is very much a part of her identity (rather than something that annihilates it) and also that she is a helpful and *valued* member of the team as they search for their friend, Nemo.

In 2006, Sarah Polley attempted to take a different approach, when she directed *Away from Her*, in which we are told the story of the later years of a couple named Fiona (who has dementia) and Grant. The story is different because it tries to focus upon the present relationship between the two main characters, with dementia being a part of their larger story, rather than the predominant focus. We are not told what, if anything, Fiona used to do for work (although she is presented as being an intelligent and vibrant woman in her pre-dementia days), and whilst there are brief moments of flashback for Grant, the main body of the film takes place in the present. Davis Basting writes, "director Sarah Polley focuses on the now, which is like an alien planet on which we must learn not to look into the future for anything – narrative meaning, progress, or hope."[32] We watch as Fiona teaches Grant how to appreciate the present moment, which enables the couple to make new connections with one another from the different neurological perspectives in which they find themselves. Davis Basting writes, "On a walk with Grant, Fiona bends down to look at a bright yellow flower and laughs. 'When I turn away, I forget yellow. Yellow is new every time. There's something delicious in oblivion,' she marvels."[33] However, although the film makes many attempts to avoid the typical tragic plotline, there is still a sense of tragedy within the story. Fiona moves to a care home and appears to lose all memory of her husband Grant, as she begins a new relationship with a fellow resident named Aubrey. At this, Grant is crestfallen and begins a relationship with Aubrey's wife. At the climax of the film, there is a final moment of lucidity, in which Fiona appears to recognise Grant as her husband once again, before the credits roll and we are left to wonder what might happen next. *Away from Her* makes an attempt to avoid painting the memory loss experience as a tragedy, whilst also going some way to frame a realistic account of the memory loss experience from the viewpoint of Grant. However, there have been other artistic attempts since that have attempted to offer an account of the memory loss experience from the viewpoint of the person living with memory loss themselves.

One of the more successful examples of attempts to represent the memory loss experience from the perspective of the person living with memory loss comes from *The Father* (2012), a play by Florian Zeller, which was later adapted for film.[34] The play tries to show how it might feel to live with memory loss by placing the reader (or audience member) inside the head of the protagonist, an elderly man called André who is living with dementia. We are invited to peep through André's narrowed eyes as he struggles to adapt to the changing status of his brain, which leads to feelings of extreme disorientation, confusion, and a belief that he is being misunderstood. The play follows André in the later stages of his dementia, as he tries to make sense of his living environment (at the beginning of the play he is living in Anne's flat, and by the end of the play he is living in a care home), his care arrangements, and (what he believes is) his daughter, Anne's, changing relationship status:

> It's been going on for some time. Strange things going on around us. Haven't you noticed? There was this man claiming this wasn't my flat. A really unsympathetic looking man. A bit like your husband. Only worse. In my flat, you understand what I'm saying? It's the best yet. Don't you think? In my flat. He told me...But...This is my flat, isn't it? Mm? Anne...This is my flat?[35]

Slips of time and tongue are presented at first as reality, and we gradually learn that much of the happenings within the play are, in fact, tricks of André's mind. Zeller achieves this by using a number of theatrical devices, including the use of two characters named, Man and Woman, who fulfil multiple roles and often appear in the place of other characters from the play, including André's daughter Anne and her husband, who is sometimes called James and sometimes called Paul. Zeller also uses a range of simple theatrical staging techniques, such as this example from the beginning of scene three: "*Simultaneously, the same room and a different room. Some furniture has disappeared: as the scenes proceed, the set sheds certain elements, until it becomes an empty, neutral space.*"[36]

The Father is an ambitious and powerful attempt to represent the memory loss experience from the perspective of the person who is living with memory loss, whilst also providing a sympathetic account of the challenges of caring for someone who is living with memory loss, in the character of Anne. However, whilst effective, the play is a work of fiction, and I will now look to pieces of work that endeavour to represent the real-life experiences of members of the memory loss community.

In his chapter, 'Dementia and the language of aging', Martin Halliwell discusses the socio-cultural background of memory loss in the context of literature.[37] Halliwell comments that whilst the 1990s saw several first person attempts at documenting the disease by people who were living with memory loss (two such examples are *Living the Labyrinth* (1993) by Diana Friel McGown and *Show me the way to go home* (1996) by Larry Rose, both of whom were diagnosed with early-onset Alzheimer's when in their 50s), most accounts of the disease are written by the child of the sufferer and the focus tends to spotlight the impact of the disease upon the child of the person who is living with memory loss, rather than the person themselves.[38,39] In this literature, the voice of the person who is living with memory loss eventually falls silent. This pursuit to obtain an authentic representation of the memory loss experience has been attempted across multiple creative disciplines, including several musical examples that attempt to give a voice to the memory loss community. One such example is *The Sky Begins to Change.*[40]

Interlude: *The Sky Begins to Change*

The Sky Begins to Change is a piece of music that was commissioned by Live Music Now in 2017 and was created by composer, musician, and author, Kerry Andrew. The work combines words from participants (most of whom were living with memory loss) from eighteen care homes in the North of England, with Andrew's own voice and the voices of K'antu ensemble, as well as a selection of folk instruments. When discussing the commission, Andrew writes:

> The piece was a very specific commission from the organisation Live Music Now - who wanted a piece that used their Live Music Now musicians in care home settings, and drawing on material recorded/sourced from the care home participants to create a live/recorded/video piece including my voice and the LMN ensemble K'antu.[41]

But whilst the commission itself presented clear parameters for Andrew to work within, on her personal ambition for the project, she comments, "Creatively, I wanted to make something that was very sympathetic to the elderly participants' voices, putting them and their words/stories first. An audio portrait of them and their lives."[42] The piece is beautifully composed and expertly performed (Andrew being an esteemed composer with a voice that veers in and out of otherness) but, other than a few moments of background noise and a short blues improvisation by one of the participants, the voices of the participants themselves cannot be heard; we only hear their words as spoken and sung in Andrew's voice. Unfortunately, although beautiful to listen to, this ventriloquism (although it is difficult to know whose hand is inside whom) of the participants' borrowed stories damages Andrew's attempt to create a piece of artwork that offers the authentic viewpoint of the participants. In removing their voices from the recording, Andrew's prosthetic representation of the voices of the people living with memory loss means that their voices fall silent, which leads to the question of the value of those voices.

In an attempt to understand why the use of Andrew's own voice was a condition of the commission, I spoke with Douglas Noble from Live Music Now.[43] He said that he wanted to communicate, "something of the dementia living experience to a wider population through the creative process" and that he wanted to, "produce something [that was] really high quality."[44,45] What he didn't want, was to produce what people might call a "nice little…community project."[46] In other words, when designing the parameters of the commission, Noble hoped to add value to the piece of music by using Andrew's voice, rather than the voices of the participants. In his eyes, Andrew's voice made the piece "really high quality" and if the voices of the participants themselves had been used, the final product might have been received as a "nice little…community project," which is what Noble was trying to avoid.[47,48] What Noble's justification for this directive suggests is that the voice itself is a mere vehicle for meaning, rather than something that is of equal, if not more importance than the words themselves. As Mladen Dolar writes in his book, *A Voice and Nothing More*, "[The voice is] what Lacan called, *objet petit a*" meaning *the unattainable object of desire*.[49,50] When we use our own mouths, teeth, and tongues to speak the words of others, we lose the unique otherness of the object of the voice, and the meaning of those words change. There are more words to be heard here from theological, Augustinian and Freudian perspectives, but, for now, my focus must remain on further modifications that were made to *The Sky Begins to Change,* as it was not only the voices of the participants that were removed, but, also, some of the words themselves.

When asked how effectively she felt she had created an authentic representation of the participants in the project, Andrew said, "it's not a true, whole reflection of them and their entire character - in fact, I was asked to take a portion of the piece out, because it included a little anger/distress/confusion of one participant over some memories. One of the partners asked for it to be removed so that it only includes nice memories! I'd have preferred to have something more rounded in, but I understood."[51] When I asked Noble about this, he said that the request to remove that part of the piece came from the senior management team from one of the care providers that they were working with on the commission, and that, although he also felt that leaving that moment in would have "enhanced its truth," it was necessary to take it out in order to "get the piece out" which was "touch and go at that point."[52,53,54] When asked about this in a later interview, Andrew said that she felt that taking out that section of the composition felt like she was, "erasing truth."[55]

The Sky Begins to Change is illustrative of the way in which we are restricted by the formula of "self = memory" and "loss of memory = loss of self."[56] Even when the aim is to offer a voice and authentic representation of a person living with memory loss, we are met with obstacles, all of which are underpinned by those simple formulas. In this case, and from the perspective of the commissioner, the voices of the participants had lost value due to their memory loss, and, even though the participants still had the ability to use their voices, that was taken away in an enforced act of loss of self in order to add value to the composition, and the words that were removed were taken out because they did not fit with the 'happy memory loss experience' that the care homes were trying to sell to the participants and their families. What is missing in *The Sky Begins to Change* is an understanding of the value and worth of the silenced voices, because, as Dolar has it, "not all voices are heard, and perhaps the most intrusive and compelling are the unheard voices."[57] However, perhaps what is most worrying is that the participants were not only denied the opportunity to use their own voices and their own words but were even denied the right to express the experience of a normal range of human emotions (anger, distress, confusion) as is expected of a person with a normal, healthy human brain.

End of interlude

The Sky Begins to Change provides a useful demonstration of the challenges that arise when trying to create a representation of the memory loss experience, which is due to the lack of value that is placed on the memory loss state. Again, I am reminded of Davis Basting's, "self = memory" and "loss of memory = loss of self" which, she argues, "inform so much of our thinking about people with dementia and determine how we care for them" and whilst I have shown how this Sacksian legacy has influenced both cultural perceptions and artistic representations of the memory loss state, I would now like to take a moment to consider how this perspective influences the way that we care for people who are living with memory loss, by looking at music therapy practices.[58]

Interlude: music therapy practices

Sacks' work on music and the brain was hugely influential in the development of music therapy practices. In *Musicophilia: Tales of Music and the Brain*, which was first published in 2007, Sacks writes, "The aim of music therapy in people with dementia...seeks to address the emotions, cognitive powers, thoughts, and memories, the surviving 'self' of the patient, to stimulate these and bring them to the fore."[59,60] I asked Dr Ming Hung Hsu (a senior research fellow at The Cambridge Institute for Music Therapy Research with a particular interest in using music therapy with people living with memory loss) what a typical music therapy session would involve. He said that, typically, "a music therapist would provide a selection of handheld percussion instruments...and the person with memory loss can just pick up any of these instruments so they can interact with the music therapist without using any words."[61] He then went on to say that the therapist would then decide whether to, "improvise freely, or... use a more song-based approach."[62] On the songs themselves, Hsu comments that the therapist will play, "familiar songs, or the songs that the client prefers," before explaining that the aim of doing this is to, "use the songs to induce some interaction and sometimes these songs can stimulate memory recalls. The client may start to talk about past memories, so talking is obviously involved as well."[63,64] To put it simply, what happens in a conventionally successful music therapy session for a person living with memory loss is the following: a therapist plays some familiar songs in the hope that they will stimulate the brain and 'wake the person up' (as in the famous case of Henry wakes up).[65] This hopefully brings the person into a short period of lucidity, during which they are able to talk to the therapist about the memories that the song or piece of music has reminded them of. There is so much more to unpack here, not least about the relationship between mourning and nostalgia and the Derridean theory of 'forgetting well', but for now, our focus must remain on Sacks. It is easy to see how Sacks' thinking on the necessity of reclaiming a pre-memory loss identity ("We must 'recollect' ourselves") has infiltrated the design of this therapeutic approach.[66] Success in these sessions is achieved when the person living with memory loss connects to their memories from the past, which is an ethos which underpins the cultural narrative to which we have become so accustomed. As highlighted in my interview with Hsu, the problem with current music therapy models is that they support the Sacksian narrative that memory loss is a tragic thing which equates to a loss of identity, and that the only way to reclaim a pre-memory loss identity (which Sacks believes is absolutely necessary if one is to preserve any sense of self) is to try to find a way to push the person back into their pre-memory loss identity by connecting them with their memories from the past. This idea is echoed in many examples of music therapy research, with one such example being conducted by researcher, Ayelet Dassa in 2018.

In Dassa's work, "'Opening Our Time Capsule' – Creating an Individualized Music and Other Memory Cues Database to Promote Communication Between Spouses and People With Dementia During Visits to a Nursing Home," the objective was to, "help alleviate caregivers' burden during visiting hours, by promoting communication opportunities. The program included the creation of an individualized database using personal music and photos that present life episodes."[67,68] This work is indicative of research concerning the therapeutic benefits of musical engagement for people living with memory loss, as it not only supports the Sacksian narrative of the need to 'push someone back' into a previous identity (and the 'success' of the research is judged on whether or not this has been achieved) but it also focuses on the feelings and wellbeing of the caregiver, rather than the participant who is living with memory loss. On her findings, Dassa writes, "All [caregiving participants] reported that using the individualized database helped them to find ways to communicate with their partners, relive shared past experiences, and alleviate the stress and feelings of disconnect during visits."[69] However, there is no mention of the impact that the musical engagement had upon research participants who were living with memory loss during the study, nor is there an understanding of the way in which the use of memory cues can be disorientating and upsetting for a person who is living with memory loss.

When I asked Hsu about the next steps for music therapy research, he said that we must, "develop and tailor this therapy to suit the needs of this population" and begin to work beyond the session-based approach which is a result of the therapy being a "psychosocial…or non-pharmacological intervention [with a close relation to] psychotherapy."[70,71] He commented that there is a need for there to be a legacy to the therapy after the session has finished, so that patients are advised how to continue with the therapy when the therapist is not there, as is already the case with therapies such as speech and language therapy and physiotherapy. Hsu also notes that, whilst he was not aware of any music therapies that directly involve joint participation between a person living with memory loss and a friend or family member, when a friend or family member (in one particular case, a person's wife) did join in with a session, it was, "extremely beneficial to the music therapist," and that it was also a positive experience for the wife, because she was able to see her husband, "enjoying the music."[72,73] There is a move towards this approach within the field, with one example being that of the work of Ray and Götell in their study, "The Use of Music and Music Therapy in Ameliorating Depression Symptoms and Improving Well-being in Nursing Home Residents With Dementia," in which music therapists trained care workers to carry out musical engagement tasks as part of a wider care programme without the need for the presence of a music therapist, and the result was positive.[74] On the study, Ray and Götell reported that "Music activities designed by music therapists and facilitated by CNAs [certified nursing assistants] may help sustain the reduction of depression symptoms and improve wellbeing in nursing home residents with moderate to severe dementia."[75] This is in line with Hsu's thinking for the next steps in music therapy practices, and I will return to Hsu's comments in the conclusion of this book, when I will use the data that I have collected to make suggestions for future therapy practices, which, as he says, need to be tailored to, "suit the needs of the population."[76] An illuminating step towards this is to examine the way in which the population is starting to evolve, through the pioneering testimony of dementia campaigner, Dr Wendy Mitchell.

End of interlude

Wendy Mitchell

Wendy Mitchell was diagnosed with young-onset dementia in July 2014 at the age of fifty-eight. She is the author of three books; *Somebody I Used to Know* (2018), *What I Wish People Knew about Dementia from Someone Who Knows* (2022), and *One Last Thing: How to Live with the End in Mind* (2023), and she also writes a blog named, *Which Me and I today?* in which she talks openly and honestly about the memory loss experience.[77,78,79,80] Fuelled by her shock of the lack of awareness about her disease when she was first diagnosed, Mitchell campaigns widely in order to raise awareness and offer a more positive perspective of memory loss, because, in her words, "nothing is impossible even for someone with brain disease."[81]

In *What I Wish People Knew about Dementia, from Someone Who Knows,* Mitchell writes, "Everyone has their challenges, mine just happens to be dementia."[82] Mitchell's writing goes some way to normalise the dementia experience. Her memory loss means that she faces many practical challenges in her daily life, and she talks about these candidly. However, Mitchell focuses much attention upon the challenges that she faces which are a direct result of the cultural perception of the memory loss experience. On artistic representations, Mitchell writes, "Dementia is represented more often in arts and fiction these days, though accurate portrayals are not always found in books and television, and writers and screenwriters can often rely on clichés to get their messages across to audiences quickly."[83] I am reminded here of the cliché of the tragic hero narrative, and, as a member of the memory loss community, it is understandable that Mitchell is disheartened by the repetition of a single plot line that attempts to represent the entire memory loss community. Mitchell goes on to say, "Film and media producers do not merely set out to provide an accurate description of dementia. They have an interest in obtaining a certain impact, in providing entertainment, suspense and dramatic effect. They allow themselves a certain artistic license."[84] The ethical question of artistic license when one is given the responsibility of representing a group of people to which they do not belong is brought into sharp focus in this context. Even in *The Sky Begins to Change*, in which a sensitive portrayal of the participants' lives was the aim, artistic license was used to determine the use of voices and words that were used, which silenced the participants' voices and (even in the eye of the composer) damaged the truth of the piece. On this, Mitchell writes, "But each of us has a responsibility that our portrayals of others are accurate, balanced and respectful, or at least that's what those of us with dementia ask."[85]

On the importance of language and the way in which the memory loss community is treated and represented, Mitchell writes, "I often think now about how important the doctor's choice of words and use of language is when speaking to patients."[86] She also speaks of "how health professionals overlook the person sitting in front of them, discussing them as a 'sufferer', writing them off with their diagnosis."[87] Mitchell notes that this negative language that is used by health professionals is also problematic within representations of memory loss in the media. She writes, "the media don't help either, always referring to 'dementia sufferers', and how dispiriting the images are, too, such as the photographs of bed-bound old ladies that I'd first found when I'd first googled dementia."[88] Here, Mitchell is highlighting the impact that the Sacksian repetition of negative words (based on the neurological perspective that normal brain = good, and changed brain = bad) continues to have on the way in which we view and treat the memory loss community. However, whilst Mitchell's critique of both cultural representations of the memory loss experience and the language that is used when talking to, and about people who are living with memory loss, she is beginning to move the discussion in a new direction, in which she focusses on explaining how the memory loss experience *feels*.

On the 3 October 2022, I interviewed Wendy Mitchell about her first book, *Somebody I Used to Know*.[89,90] Just as she does in her book, she talked at length about the negative impact of the catastrophic language used by health professionals and the media when talking about the memory loss experience. However, we also discussed how her memory loss diagnosis has an impact on other matters, such as her identity, relationships, and the way in which she adapts to the changing status of her brain in order to continue to engage with creative practices. On identity, I asked:

"***Sam:*** So obviously you have your wonderful blog, *Which me am I today?*, and you make quite a lot of references in your book about having a new identity. You say, "But now there's this new me"[91] and you have these letters to your former self where you talk about yourself in the third person. And I'm interested to know whether you feel as though you have a new identity now that you have dementia.

Wendy: I'm still the same me on the outside. I don't feel the same me on the inside. I feel like I look at the old me, and have her as a companion to ask, 'What shall I do now? What would you do?' I think in my book I said that all my daughters now call me this gregarious alien, because they are shocked at the person I've become. My personality has changed so much. I was so private. I don't think I was shy. I just liked my own company and my own being. But now I talk to people like you quite freely. I would never have done that."[92]

Here, Mitchell goes some way to explain the thinking behind the title of her blog (*Which me am I today?*), whilst also suggesting that it might be helpful to think of people who are living with memory loss as having multiple identities.[93] In introducing the idea of having a second, or 'new' identity, Mitchell places herself in the present and future space, which opens up the possibility for the new identity to be one that could be thought of as having value, even when the circumstances mean that her 'first' identity might be thought of as lost, due to the loss of her memory. When I then asked her about the way in which her memory loss has an impact on her relationships with people, she said this:

"***Sam:*** You write in your book, "I arrive at the gates and spot someone waving at me. They seem vaguely familiar and when we meet, they tell me it isn't the first time."[94] I was wondering if you could describe what that feeling feels like.

Wendy: That happens daily. I've just been to the village tea and toast morning to sell my calendars. People come and hug me and I haven't a clue who they are. I know I know them because they're so warm and comforting. I haven't a clue what their name is or anything, so it's the emotional feeling you get. I can have emotional feelings where I know I don't like the person, even though I don't know why, and I react differently to them. If someone says, "Ohh morning, Wendy!," and gives me a hug, because I feel that warmth from them. I feel an icy cold from someone that I know I don't like for some reason, or maybe they've hurt me, or maybe something's happened that means that I don't like them. It's the emotions that take over any form of identity."[95]

Here, Mitchell is hinting at her memory loss state having an uncanny emotional intelligence that compensates for the fact that she struggles to recall people that she has previously met. Once again, by explaining what the memory loss status feels like, she is able to suggest that, although different, the memory loss brain might be thought of as an intelligent brain that can hold value. I also asked

Mitchell about the potentially therapeutic benefits of engaging in certain creative practices:

"***Sam:*** And obviously you're a writer and a photographer, and you write about how you play Scrabble and you read short stories. You also just mentioned painting pebbles. Are there any other creative practices that you find particularly helpful?

Wendy: I have a routine in the morning where I play lots of games, but always without the sound. I can't cope with any sound being on the mic. It distracts me. Everything is in silence, which again, people don't like silence. They find that very difficult. Sometimes people think I'm doing nothing on my iPad because there's no noise, but I might have done, I don't know, five or six games of Scrabble or something like that. So people have to learn to appreciate silence, because our brains can't cope with two things coming in at once. Music is wonderful. Just music. Can't be music and conversation. It doesn't work. We can't do two things at once."[96]

Again, Mitchell sheds light on the memory loss experience by explaining, not only how she believes her brain works, but also the impact that multiple sensory inputs have upon her ability to process thought. She is also explaining how a very simple adaptation (turning the sound off her iPad, for example) means that she is still able to benefit from and enjoy engaging in a range of creative practices.

Mitchell is ambitious in the way in which she attempts to challenge the cultural perception of the memory loss state, even to the point of describing her Alzheimer's disease as "a gift."[97] In educating others in how the memory loss experience feels to her, she hopes to begin to shape opinions, practices, and developments in research, whilst also positioning people who are living with memory loss in a position of value in the future space. This is in direct opposition to the Sacksian narrative that (as I have demonstrated using the examples given in this chapter) has had an overpowering impact on the way in which we currently think about, creatively represent, and care for the memory loss community. At the beginning of this chapter, I wrote that I wanted to explore whether a better understanding of the memory loss experience might shift the current perception of the value of the memory loss brain, and Mitchell's work demonstrates how it is possible to disrupt cultural perceptions of value by taking an approach which is fuelled by inclusion, accessibility, and understanding. In the chapter that follows this, I share five case studies which are taken from an interpretative phenomenological analysis investigation in which I aimed to gather data that sheds further light on the memory loss experience, whilst also supporting the ethos of this research; that an identity changed by memory loss is different, not less. But first, please read, hear, and listen to *Spin* (Figure 2.1), an experimental conflict for mouths and bodies that uses the

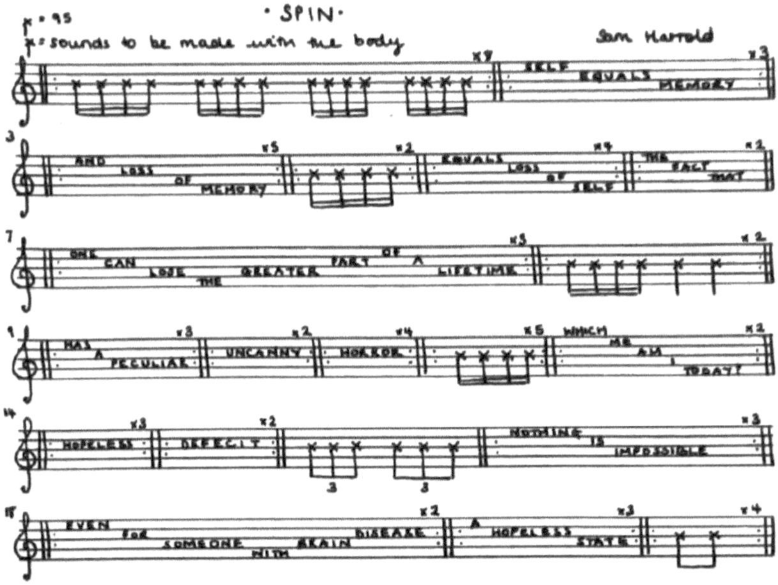

Figure 2.1 Excerpt from *Spin*, taken from Appendix B. www.routledge.com/9781041072652

Please go to www.routledge.com/9781041072652 to listen to this and to read the score.

polarising speech fragments from this literature to encourage a new approach to listening and seeing.

Notes

1 Davis Basting, A. (2009) *Forget Memory.* Baltimore: The John Hopkins University Press. P24.
2 Davis Basting, A. (2009) P24.
3 Davis Basting, A. (2009) P181.
4 Davis Basting, A. (2009) P181.
5 Davis Basting, A. (2009) P181.
6 Davis Basting, A. (2009) P181.
7 Sacks, O. (2011) The Man Who Mistook His Wife for a Hat. London: Picador.
8 Tougaw, J. (2018) *The Elusive Brain: Literary Experiments in the Age of Neuroscience.* United States of America: Yale University Press.
9 Tougaw, J. (2018) P42.
10 Tougaw, J. (2018) P41.
11 Sacks, O. (2011).
12 Sacks, O. (2011).
13 Menaker, D. (2019) Oliver Sacks's Final, Posthumous Work [online] Available at: https://www.nytimes.com/2019/04/30/books/review/everything-in-its-place-oliver-sacks.html [Accessed: July 5th, 2024]
14 Sacks, O. (2011) P25.

15 Sacks, O. (2011) P43.
16 Sacks, O. (2011) P25.
17 Sacks, O. (2011) P25.
18 Sacks, O. (2011) P36.
19 Sacks, O. (2011) P37.
20 Sacks, O. (2011) P42.
21 Sacks, O. (2011) P42.
22 Sacks, O. (2011) P91.
23 Sacks, O. (2011) P117.
24 Davis Basting, A. (2009)
25 Davis Basting, A. (2009) P24.
26 Davis Basting, A. (2009) P40.
27 Davis Basting, A. (2009) P40.
28 Ronald Reagan Presidential Library and Museum, (2022) *Reagan's Letter Announcing his Alzheimer's Diagnosis.* [online] Available at: https://www.reaganlibrary.gov/reagans/ronald-reagan/reagans-letter-announcing-his-alzheimers-diagnosis?msclkid=fbab5c95cf9011ec9d60467875ab43b0 [Accessed: May 9th, 2022] [Accessed: May the 9th, 2022]
29 Ronald Reagan Presidential Library and Museum, (2022)
30 Davis Basting, A. (2009) P41.
31 Davis Basting, A. (2009) P41.
32 Davis Basting, A. (2009) P48.
33 Davis Basting, A. (2009) P48.
34 Zeller, F. (2015) *The Mother and The Father.* (Trans. From French by C. Hampton), London: Faber & Faber.
35 Zeller, F. (2015) P100.
36 Zeller, F. (2015) P101.
37 Halliwell, M. (2017) 'Dementia and the Language of Aging', in *The Voices of Mental Health: Medicine, Politics and American Culture, 1970–2000.* New Brunswick: Rutgers University Press, pp. 97–122.
38 Halliwell, M. (2017) P114.
39 Halliwell, M. (2017) P114.
40 YouTube (2022) *Live Music Now – The Sky Begins To Change.* [online] Available at: https://www.youtube.com/watch?v=0HeHypcDPgs [Accessed: May 9th, 2022]
41 Appendix F. www.routledge.com/9781041072652
42 Appendix F. www.routledge.com/9781041072652
43 Appendix G. www.routledge.com/9781041072652
44 Appendix G. www.routledge.com/9781041072652
45 Appendix G. www.routledge.com/9781041072652
46 Appendix G. www.routledge.com/9781041072652
47 Appendix G. www.routledge.com/9781041072652
48 Appendix G. www.routledge.com/9781041072652
49 Dolar, Mladen (2006) *A Voice and Nothing More.* Massachusetts: The MIT Press.
50 Dolar, Mladen (2006) P11.
51 Appendix F. www.routledge.com/9781041072652
52 Appendix G. www.routledge.com/9781041072652
53 Appendix G. www.routledge.com/9781041072652
54 Appendix G. www.routledge.com/9781041072652
55 Appendix H. www.routledge.com/9781041072652
56 Davis Basting, A. (2009) P24.
57 Dolar, Mladen (2006) P14.
58 Davis Basting, A. (2009) P24.

59 Sacks, O. (2007) *Musicophilia: Tales of Music and the Brain.* London: Picador.
60 Sacks, O. (2007) PP336–337.
61 Appendix I. www.routledge.com/9781041072652
62 Appendix I. www.routledge.com/9781041072652
63 Appendix I. www.routledge.com/9781041072652
64 Appendix I. www.routledge.com/9781041072652
65 YouTube (2022) *(Original) Man in Nursing Home Reacts to Hearing Music from His Era.* [online] Available at: https://www.youtube.com/watch?v=fyZQf0p73QM&t=43s [Accessed: May 9th, 2022]
66 Sacks, O. (2011) P117.
67 Dassa, A. (2018) "Opening Our Time Capsule" – Creating an individualized music and other memory cues database to promote communication between spouses and people with dementia during visits to a nursing home. *Frontiers of Medicine,* Volume 5, Issue 215. PP1–7. DOI: 10.3389/fmed.2018.00215.
68 Dassa, A. (2018) P1.
69 Dassa, A. (2018) P1.
70 Appendix I. www.routledge.com/9781041072652
71 Appendix I. www.routledge.com/9781041072652
72 Appendix I. www.routledge.com/9781041072652
73 Appendix I. www.routledge.com/9781041072652
74 Ray, K. D., Götell, E. (2018) The Use of Music and Music Therapy in Ameliorating Depression Symptoms and Improving Well-being in Nursing Home Residents With Dementia. *Frontiers of Medicine,* Volume 5, Issue 287. PP1–6. DOI: 10.3389/fmed.2018.00287.
75 Ray, K.D., Götell, E. (2018) P1.
76 Appendix I. www.routledge.com/9781041072652
77 Mitchell, W. (2019)
78 Mitchell, W. (2022) *What I Wish People Knew about Dementia from Someone Who Knows.* London: Bloomsbury Publishing.
79 Mitchell, W. (2023) *One Last Thing: How to live with the end in mind.* London: Bloomsbury Publishing.
80 Mitchell, W (2022) *Which me am I today?* [online] Available at: https://whichmeamitoday.wordpress.com/blog/ [Accessed: May 9th, 2022]
81 Mitchell, W. (2019) P273.
82 Mitchell, W. (2022) P73.
83 Mitchell, W. (2022) P101.
84 Mitchell, W. (2022) P101.
85 Mitchell, W. (2022) P102.
86 Mitchell, W. (2019) P170.
87 Mitchell, W. (2019) PP113–114.
88 Mitchell, W. (2019) P173.
89 Appendix J. www.routledge.com/9781041072652
90 Mitchell, W. (2019)
91 Mitchell, W. (2019) P288.
92 Appendix J. www.routledge.com/9781041072652
93 Mitchell, W (2022) [Accessed: May 9th, 2022]
94 Mitchell, W. (2019) P252.
95 Appendix J. www.routledge.com/9781041072652
96 Appendix J. www.routledge.com/9781041072652
97 Mitchell, W. (2019) P32.

Bibliography

Dassa, A. (2018) "Opening Our Time Capsule" – Creating an individualized music and other memory cues database to promote communication between spouses and people with dementia during visits to a nursing home. *Frontiers of Medicine*, Volume 5, Issue 215. PP1–7. DOI: 10.3389/fmed.2018.00215.

Davis Basting, A. (2009) *Forget Memory*. Baltimore: The John Hopkins University Press.

Dolar, Mladen (2006) *A Voice and Nothing More*. Massachusetts: The MIT Press.

Halliwell, M. (2017) 'Dementia and the Language of Aging', in *The Voices of Mental Health: Medicine, Politics and American Culture, 1970–2000*. New Brunswick: Rutgers University Press, pp. 97–122.

Menaker, D. (2019) Oliver Sacks's Final, Posthumous Work [online] Available at: https://www.nytimes.com/2019/04/30/books/review/everything-in-its-place-oliver-sacks.html [Accessed: July 5th, 2024]

Mitchell, W. (2019) *Somebody I Used to Know*. London: Bloomsbury Publishing.

Mitchell, W. (2022) *What I Wish People Knew about Dementia from Someone Who Knows*. London: Bloomsbury Publishing.

Mitchell, W. (2022) *Which me am I today?* [online] Available at: https://whichmeamitoday.wordpress.com/blog/ [Accessed: May 9th, 2022]

Mitchell, W. (2023) *One Last Thing: How to Live with the End in Mind*. London: Bloomsbury Publishing.

Ray, K. D., Götell, E. (2018) The use of music and music therapy in ameliorating depression symptoms and improving well-being in nursing home residents with dementia. *Frontiers of Medicine*, Volume 5, Issue 287. PP1–6. DOI: 10.3389/fmed.2018.00287.

Ronald Reagan Presidential Library and Museum (2022) *Reagan's Letter Announcing his Alzheimer's Diagnosis*. [online] Available at: https://www.reaganlibrary.gov/reagans/ronald-reagan/reagans-letter-announcing-his-alzheimers-diagnosis?msclkid=fbab5c95cf9011ec9d60467875ab43b0 [Accessed: May 9th, 2022]

Sacks, O. (2007) *Musicophilia: Tales of Music and the Brain*. London: Picador.

Sacks, O. (2011) *The Man Who Mistook His Wife for a Hat*. London: Picador.

Tougaw, J. (2018) *The Elusive Brain: Literary Experiments in the Age of Neuroscience*. United States of America: Yale University Press.

YouTube (2022) *Live Music Now - The Sky Begins to Change*. [Online] Available at: https://www.youtube.com/watch?v=0HeHypcDPgs [Accessed: May 9th, 2022]

YouTube (2022) *(Original) Man In Nursing Home Reacts to Hearing Music From His Era*. [online] Available at: https://www.youtube.com/watch?v=fyZQf0p73QM&t=43s [Accessed: May 9th, 2022]

Zeller, F. (2015) *The Mother and The Father*. (Trans. From French by C. Hampton), London: Faber & Faber.

Chapter 3

Five strange stories

A note on the research process and the nursing home environment

As I mentioned in the introduction to this book, my research design challenges traditional definitions of ethnographic inquiry in that it took place in the uncanny environment of a nursing home. It was not possible for the sessions with primary participants to take place elsewhere for health reasons, so all sessions from that particular participant group took place within the strange world of the nursing home environment.

When discussing her aim when running the nursing home, the manager at the nursing home acknowledged how unnatural the environment was.[1] She said, "What we want, I suppose, is to make everybody happy and we can't. We want everyone to have a happy life and to be… But this is an unnatural environment. This is a nursing home. It's not their own home."[2] When asked how she went about easing the transition from home to nursing home for service users who were living with memory loss, she said, "We get the past history which is very helpful. Photographs, family photographs, you know, and, what else? If the family could bring in important items that are meaningful to them for their bedrooms so that their surroundings look a bit familiar. So, we have people who don't leave their room and we kind of put as much around the room that will remind them of their home. Although they know it's not their home, at least they'll see things that look familiar, a familiar blanket, that kind of thing. You know, it's just something that they might touch and think, 'Oh yes, I had this in my previous place' wherever that was."[3]

Unfortunately, this attempt to make something other an *another* merely exacerbates the strange feeling of the new environment, and this sensation of defamiliarisation and distancing is agitated further by the general sensory environment of the nursing home. Upon entry, one is immediately confronted with the tinny sounds of multiple music players that work in semi-phase as they spit out strange songs of recent and recognisable pasts. These are accompanied by clinking china cups, out-of-tune (always flat) doorbells, earth-shaking alarms, and occasional distant and barely there calls for help. This uncomfortable sound world is joined by a persistent wave of clashing food smells, the glare of hot, bright television screens, and the

DOI: 10.4324/9781003639657-3

scattered ubiquitous gaze of peculiar glass eyes which watch from the worn faces of (un)familiar dolls and teddy bears. Occasionally, a goat or horse will appear wearing a nappy, in the name of pet therapy. Nursing homes are the uncanniest of environments. For someone who is already living a life of the vaguely familiar due to their memory loss experience, it is easy to see how disorientating the nursing home environment must feel. I am reminded here not only of Freud's uncanny but also of Brecht's verfremdungseffekt, and during my study, I witnessed the effects of estrangement that are felt and experienced by people who live in these unhomely homes.

All data that I have collected from primary participants is located within the world of the nursing home, and whilst the nursing home setting challenges the use of the word ethnographic in the study design, the nursing home experience is an integral part of the experiences of each primary participant and is, therefore, an integral part of the human data that I have collected. I acknowledge this in detail in Chapter 4.

This IPA research project was carried out rigorously, ethically, and creatively. Every carefully made design choice was made in line with the IPA methodology, and the wellbeing of the participants was prioritised when making every decision throughout the process. I carried out the research with kindness and integrity and the feedback that I gathered from the participants at the end of the study is overwhelmingly positive. Although this approach is not yet commonly used alongside creative practice, the flexible framework of the methodology allowed me to design the research to suit my own creative strengths and experience, which enhanced both the participatory experience for the participants and also the quality of the data collected. The result of this research design is a most unusual and enchanting data set which provides an important, valuable, and timely insight into the memory loss experience. Before I share my findings, I offer, *Strange World* (Figure 3.1), an environmental sound chance piece which was composed in response to the unpleasant and over-stimulating sound world of the nursing home environment.

Five strange stories

The experience of carrying out the fieldwork for this project was extraordinary. Over the period of two particularly rainy months, I sat next to the final beds and chairs of ten strange strangers (A memory: "You must run and scream!") as they shared the stories of their lives and their deaths with me. Their bodies (which were partially concealed by identical linens) were collapsing, folding, and spoiling in stop motion, but their soft mouths, fluttering tongues, and clacking teeth seemed impelled to speak. They told me of heavenly summers spent working on Swiss campsites in their early twenties. They told me of yellow taffeta dresses that their mothers had carefully sewn for them by hand when they were three. They told me how the butterflies in their tummy (which were still there, now frozen in taxidermy) had felt when they had played the piano in front of an audience for the first time. They told me of unusual buttons shaped like sweet sleeping foxes on warm

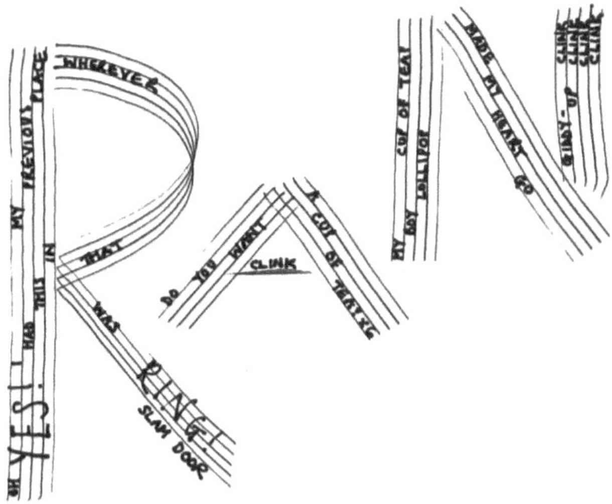
OH YES! I HAD THIS IN MY PREVIOUS PLACE
WHEREVER
THAT
WAS
RING!
SLAM DOOR
DO YOU WANT A CUP OF TEA?
CLINK
MY BOY LOLLIPOP
CUP OF TEA?
MADE MY HEART GO
GIDDY-UP
CLINK
CLINK
CLINK
CLINK

Figure 3.1 Excerpt from *Strange World*, taken from Appendix C. www.routledge.com/9781041072652

Please go to www.routledge.com/9781041072652 to listen to this and to read the score.

winter coats. They told me that a cruel ex-partner had cut off one of their fingers. They told me that when their brothers, sisters, fathers, husbands, and nieces had died it had broken their hearts, and they told me that they were not frightened of dying. Collectively, their recollections had something to do with the archival impulse to tell one's own stories. They had something to do with the work of living. They had something to do with the work of dying. And they had something to do with the uncanny. During that time, I learned more than I could hope to fit into these coming pages, partly due to the confines of my word limit but more so because much of the very otherness of these peculiar happenings is something that I am still puzzling over, and I expect to continue to do so for some time. However, what I can share at this point can be summarised thus: the memory loss experience is *strange.*

Strangeness, by very nature, is a difficult thing to define. Put simply, the word strange is used to describe something that is something else. It is the sound Edgar Allan Poe describes as having an "unearthly peculiarity" in *The Facts in the Case of M. Valdemar.*[4] It is an un-named woman who believes herself to be a reincarnated snail asking, "What was I doing in this uncalled-for-body?" in Margaret Atwood's, *Old Babes in the Wood.*[5] It is the feeling of travelling to the year 802,701 that the Time Traveller in H. G. Wells' *The Time Machine* describes as "peculiar" and "excessively unpleasant."[6,7] Strangeness is the feeling of estrangement provoked by new/old, (un)familiar places and faces. It is the impossible almost-space between the nearest and the near, and the not-quite-there sounds that linger with bitter-sweetness on the tips of our tongues. It is a piece of music that syringe-flushes out our bones, and it is a word sitting patiently in a cloud of warm breath, waiting for an ear to find its meaning. Strangeness is magical, unbearable, hidden, exposed, missing, found, lingering, vanishing, external, internal, human, and non-human. Strangeness is something else.

And now, I am going to tell these strange stories. They are stories of life, music, and words. They are stories of multiple identities, tilted senses, and ingrained environmental sounds. They are stories of final conversations, streams of unconsciousness, and *the very last thing*. The following five case studies give a rare glimpse into the curious diorama of the memory loss world; an Escher's staircase of strangely familiar feelings, memories, and moments that superimpose themselves onto the minds of people who are living with memory loss like a palimpsest.

Case study 1

Participant 9: "She can't read anymore."

I was first introduced to Participant 9, not by name, but as one of 'the three ladies in the lounge.' The lounge was one of three communal spaces in the nursing home and was small, loud, and scattered with a collection of confusing odds and ends. Among these curious things was something I have never seen before; a completely stringless (and, therefore, unbearably silent) upright piano. There was also a cushion that had a photograph of an ex-resident's grandchildren on it, an old ragdoll which was the size of a five-year-old child, and several unopened bottles of white wine. The room was awkwardly shaped, but the staff had managed to make space for about seven small brown armchairs, which had been arranged in order to provide their occupants with the best possible view of the enormous television. The finest seats in the room were the three chairs that sat in a line opposite the television, and these were reserved for the three ladies in the lounge. Participant 9 would sit in the chair on the left, Participant 8 would sit in the chair in the middle, and Participant 4 would sit in the chair on the right. Above their heads was a large mirror, onto which somebody had attached an A4 piece of paper that read, "Our Golden Girls!!!" (I wondered whether there was a significance to the three exclamation marks?) in clumsily written black ink. In front of each of the three ladies sat a brown overbed table on wheels, and those belonging to Participant 9 and Participant 8 had been decorated with artwork that had been produced during the activity sessions that took place at the nursing home. Participant 9's table had a piece of paper stuck to it, onto which someone had written her name in bubble writing. Beside her name was a drawing of a lily. Both the name and the lily had been coloured in with a red felt tip pen and the precious piece of paper had been covered completely with strips of sellotape (the edges of which were now curling and brown) in an attempt to protect it from spilled tea and biscuit crumbs. A small, multicoloured woollen pom-pom also hung from the screw that allowed the height of the table to be adjusted. The three ladies spent every day sitting in these three chairs. They sat facing forward (their tuckered necks were too tired to turn) in this side-by-side line (or was it a queue?), and although they did not appear to care for each other particularly (during one lunch time I heard Participant 4 bark, "For God's sake, just shut up and eat your potatoes!" to Participant 8), they appeared to take some comfort from the presence of each other and were reluctant to be separated.

Participant 9 was the most confused and distressed of the three ladies, which annoyed Participant 4. She was a talented knitter, and the nursing home staff had positioned a basket of plump wool and some knitting needles next to her chair. She would knit many small squares (suitable for a patchwork blanket that would never be made) during the course of each day. However, she seemed to take little comfort from this and would spend most of the day crying, and whispering, "Where am I?" and "Why am I here?" to nobody in particular. The nursing home staff would try very hard to lift her mood. They would do this by attempting to distract her with an activity such as a jigsaw puzzle, or a conversation in which they would try to change the subject. This would work for a very short amount of time, and she would briefly stop crying whilst her mind was distracted with thoughts of something else. However, after about five minutes, at the most, she would return to feeling distressed.

Although Participant 9's short-term memory was very poor, she was extremely articulate, and she seemed to enjoy the informal discussions that I had with her in the lounge. She particularly enjoyed talking about babies and young children (these conversations would make her laugh) and she was delighted when one of her granddaughters visited on one occasion, although she became especially disorientated and upset when she left. Participant 9 seemed to warm to me during my time at the nursing home and would greet me with a delayed smile and a cautious but affable "hello" each time I entered the lounge. Like many of the women I met whilst I was there, she would often reach out and take my hand whilst we were talking.

As with all participants who were living with memory loss, Participant 9 completed a life story interview for her first session.[8] In this, she was able to remember very little about her life, but she seemed to enjoy the conversation. I conducted the same interview again the following week, but before the second interview, I played her some music (Chopin's Nocturnes, Op.27: No2 in D Flat Major) in order to see if the music had an impact on the answers that she was able to give.[9] Even though the questions were the same as the questions I had asked her the previous week, she had no memory of them, so I was able to use this technique to measure the impact that listening to the music had upon our conversation. Following this, and owing to some comments that she had made about a lost love of reading due to her memory loss during the first two sessions, I decided to share a quick fiction with her during her third session.[10] This was a successful intervention for Participant 9, which I developed further in her fourth session by reading alongside her and discussing the reading together.[11] I have chosen to share the results of my time spent with Participant 9 as my first case study, as the findings are in keeping with two of my initial hypotheses that I outlined in the introduction to this book. These being that (a) whilst listening to music can induce a period of lucidity for people who are living with memory loss, this can be distressing, and (b) due to neuroplasticity, people with memory loss can continue to learn and enjoy new things.

The recording of the first session with Participant 9 is not unpleasant to listen to.[12] She is in high spirits throughout the conversation, and she can often be heard to laugh.

Participant 9: *I had a brother and sister. They were both older than me. I was the baby of the family. [She laughs] That's about all I know. [She laughs]*[13]

The most striking moment of the conversation comes at the very beginning of the conversation, when she talks about the loss of her father.

Sam: *Can you think of an event from your childhood?*
Participant 9: *No. [Pause] [Suddenly more animated] Only when I lost my daddy. That's the only thing.*[14]

This moment is interesting, not only because it is one of the very few memories that she is able to share, but also because of the way in which the sound of her voice changes when she says the words, "Only when I lost my daddy" (Figure 3.2). She sings rather than speaks these words, which is entirely different to the way in which she speaks throughout the rest of the conversation.

The celebratory, "TA-DAH!" quality of this song fragment is pulled from Participant 9's memory like a rabbit from a magician's top hat. It would seem that by attaching an upbeat rhythm and lively melody to this memory of her first experience of grief, she is able to hold onto the important memory and share it in a way that eases the pain it causes.

There is one other fact that Participant 9 can recall during our first conversation, which is the name of her two children.

Sam: *And, you said you married. Did you have children?*
Participant 9: *Yeah, I had two children. A boy and a girl.* ***** *and* ******.[15]

However, whilst she is able to recall the names of her children, she does not tell me anything about them, and she cannot tell me any details at all about her grandchildren.

Sam: *And how about grandchildren?*
Participant 9: *[She laughs] Oh gosh! I've got hundreds of them!*

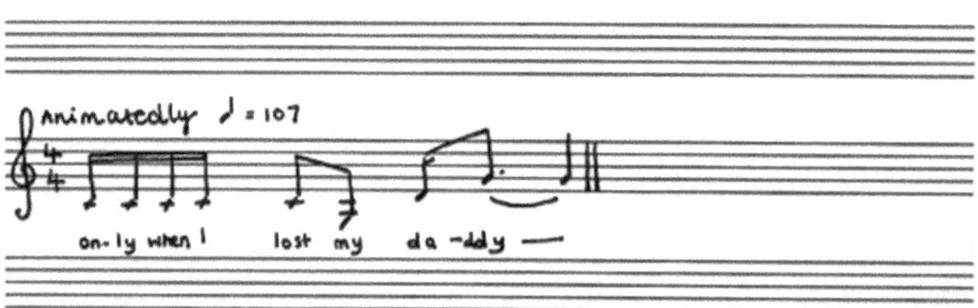

Figure 3.2 "Only when I lost my daddy."

Sam: *Have you? Goodness! How many do you have?*
Participant 9: *I don't know. I don't know how many I've got but I've got many. [She laughs] Yes, I've got quite a lot.*
Sam: *And do you like being a grandmother?*
Participant 9: *Well, I don't see them a lot. I don't really see them a great deal.*[16]

And whilst she is able to tell me that she has a religion, she is not able to tell me what it is.

Sam: *And do you have a religion?*
Participant 9: *Erm, Yes. But I don't know what you'd call it. I don't know what you'd call it.*
Sam: *Is it Church of England?*
Participant 9: *No, not Church of England.*
Sam: *Catholic?*
Participant 9: *What's the other one?*
Sam: *Catholic?*
Participant 9: *No.*
Sam: *Christianity?*
Participant 9: *Possibly that. It could be called that. Yeah.*
Sam: *And is your religion important to you?*
Participant 9: *Not very much.*[17]

These are the only pieces of information that Participant 9 is able to remember during our first session. Throughout the rest of the conversation, when I ask a question, she laughs and says that she cannot remember.

Sam: *And can you remember anything from your teenage years?*
Participant 9: *[She laughs] No, I can't remember.*
Sam: *That's OK.*
Participant 9: *I'm not very good at remembering anything.*[18]

At no point in the first session with Participant 9 does she seem distressed or upset by the fact that she can remember so little. She repeatedly describes herself as being hopeless, but she does so in a jovial manner and does not appear to be upset by the harmful language that she is using towards herself.

Sam: *And this is the last one. If you were to look back at your life and imagine it as a story, what do you think the message or the theme of the story might be?*
Participant 9: *[She laughs] It wouldn't have any story to it! No, no. [She continues to laugh]*
Sam: *Oh well, thank you so much. It's been so lovely to talk to you. Thank you so much for your time.*

Participant 9: *[Still laughing] I think I've been absolutely hopeless!*
Sam: *No, you have not.*
Participant 9: *Hopeless!*[19]

There was an enormous contrast between the first and second sessions with Participant 9. When we listened to the Chopin before the second interview began, she had a visible physical reaction. Before I played the music she was slumped in her chair, but as she listened, her spine seemed to strengthen, and she sat up. Her chin then lifted from her chest and her eyes widened and started to gleam. It was as though she had been injected with the energy of a ghost's breath, and there was a moment where she seemed to be both calm and conscious. Her plastic neck then jolted to life which allowed her head to turn, giving her new eyes the opportunity to look around the lounge. As she drank in her new surroundings, her newly formed upper body became tense, her fingernails scratched at the arms of her chair, and her eyes started to flicker and fill with tears. It looked as though she was able to see and understand her surroundings in a way that she had not been able to before, and this appeared to make her feel confused and anxious. I was not surprised by this, as I saw this reaction to listening to music happen many times when I was visiting my late grandfather. However, it never becomes less upsetting to witness, and the reaction from my own body is always the same; the hairs on the back of my neck stand on end, and I feel strangely disconnected from myself for a brief but horrifying moment.

The recording of the second session with Participant 9 is unpleasant to listen to.[20] She is very sad and quiet. The session begins like this:

Sam: *So, this is Participant number 9, session 2. OK, so can you remember an earliest memory? Do you have an earliest memory?*
Participant 9: *[Very quietly and sadly] No.*
Sam: *That's OK. And can you think of an event from your childhood that stands out to you?*
Participant 9: *I don't remember much of my childhood, no.*
Sam: *That's OK.*
Participant 9: *[Very sadly] You're going to be very disappointed in any queries with me.*[21]

This is in stark contrast to the way in which she responds at the beginning of the first session. It is as though she has more of an awareness of the loss of her memory, which she seems to find very distressing.

Sam: *And can you think of an event in your life that stands out as being particularly important to you?*
Participant 9: *Not really. I don't remember anything much. [She starts to cry and continues to do so for the rest of the interview].*[22]

She remembers far more during the second session than she did in the first. However, the pain of some of the memories are upsetting to her.

Sam: *And can you tell me a little bit about your family? Did you get married?*
Participant 9: *Ooh yes. Married my husband. ****, he was.*
Sam: *****.*
Participant 9: *Yes.*
Sam: *And what was he like?*
Participant 9: *Lovely, but he died long before... long before he should have done.*[23]

The painful memory of the untimely death of her late husband causes her a great amount of sadness. At this point in the interview Participant 9 seems to be re-experiencing the horrifying feeling of being a newly grieving widow, which she seemed completely unaware of when talking about her marriage in the first session. She is also able to tell me far more detail about her two children.

Sam: *And how about your children? Do you have children?*
Participant 9: *Oh yeah, I had two; ***** and *******. *****'s done very well for himself. ******* has really, too.*
Sam: *Mm-hmm. What do they do?*
Participant 9: *Oh, I can't even think now. ******* was a *******, and *****'s done all sorts of things that I don't even understand, but he was quite brainy.*[24]

This is the most positive moment of the conversation, and Participant 9 seems to enjoy talking about her children's achievements. However, she soon becomes very distressed when asked questions that she finds it harder to answer.

Sam: *And, can you think of somebody who's been a positive influence in your life?*
Participant 9: *[Very sadly] No.*
Sam: *And how about a negative influence? Can you think of anybody that's been a negative influence in your life?*
Participant 9: *No. My memory's practically gone.*
Sam: *That's OK. And how about television programmes? Are there any television programmes or films that you like?*
Participant 9: *No. I can't think of any. [Crying] Oh, I'm absolutely hopeless to talk to.*
Sam: *I don't think that at all.*
Participant 9: *[Still crying] I am.*[25]

Just as in session 1, Participant 9 refers to herself as being "hopeless" when she struggles to remember something. However, the difference is that in session 1 she laughs when she calls herself this, and the fact that she cannot remember very much does not seem to upset her at all. In session 2, she also describes herself as being hopeless, but this time she does this to cruelly punish herself for her memory loss. The impact of listening to the music before the second session is very clear. It provokes a period of increased physical strength and mental lucidity, in which Participant 9 is able to recall more information than she is able to recall when she has not listened to music. However, her lucidity means that she is more aware of the fact that she cannot answer every question during the second session, and this is distressing to her; it makes her feel very sad and embarrassed. Participant 9 is also able to remember painful memories during the second session (although, curiously, she fails to mention the death of her father) which she tragically relives as they find a path in which to drip-bleed into her conscious thoughts. She has successfully been pushed backwards, or 'woken up' by the music, but the impact of this upon the wellbeing of Participant 9 is overwhelmingly negative.

When the second session had finished, I stayed in the lounge to observe Participant 9. She was extremely sad and continued to cry for some time after the interview had ended. The strength in her back and neck seemed to dissolve quickly, and her body soon folded itself back into its original position. However, her eyes remained in their state of temporary aliveness, and they began to work in a panicked double time. Her pupils rapidly flashed from left to right with absolute control and no control at all, in what seemed to be an attempt to make sense of the scene change that was happening around her. Although her body was completely still, she began to look dizzy and nauseous, as though she might pass out. Somehow, in watching her, this feeling transferred to me, and I had to swallow deeply and hold onto the arms of my chair for balance. After about five minutes, she suddenly winced and squeezed her eyelids shut, as if a fast moth was flying towards her face. Then, with her eyes still closed, she let her chin fall back onto her chest, and fell asleep.

At this point in my analysis of my time with Participant 9, I am reminded of my critique of current music therapy practices, which I supported with my reading of Oliver Sacks, and also with my interview with Dr Ming Hung Hsu in Chapter 2.[26] As a reminder, in *Musicophilia: Tales of Music and the Brain*, Sacks writes, "The aim of music therapy in people with dementia...seeks to address the emotions, cognitive powers, thoughts, and memories, the surviving "self" of the patient, to stimulate these and bring them to the fore."[27,28] Hsu confirmed that this is the case, and explained that during a typical music therapy session the therapist will play, "familiar songs, or the songs that the client prefers," and that the aim of doing this is to, "use the songs to induce some interaction and sometimes these songs can stimulate memory recalls."[29,30] My concern with this approach stems from the informal observations that I made when visiting my grandfather in a care home between 2017 and 2019. During this time, and as mentioned in Chapter 1, I organised and performed at several concerts at his care home, and I also witnessed many musical activities which had been arranged by the home during times when I happened to be visiting. It is worth mentioning at this moment that my motivation for arranging the concerts, and for visiting the care home several times a week, was to spend time with my grandfather, not to observe the impact that musical engagement had upon the residents. It is also of note that as a musician of over 30 years who has played in all sorts of community settings (a folk concert series many years ago on a hospital ward for elderly people comes to mind) I did not expect to discover that listening to music could have a negative impact on anyone, and on a personal level that is still something that I am troubling over. However, I have seen many times that listening to music can stimulate a period of lucidity for someone who is living with memory loss, in which they are able to recall memories that would otherwise by forgotten. But this period of lucidity brings with it a realisation that the person has a problem with their memory, and also allows them to recall painful memories that would otherwise be buried. This, coupled with a prolonged moment of semi-clarity over their (un)familiar surroundings is distressing, as was the case in my second session with Participant 9.

After my second session with Participant 9, I spent some time reflecting on the recordings and transcriptions of the first two sessions in order to plan for the third session. I was troubled by how distressed Participant 9 had become during her second session with me, and I wanted to see if I could find a creative outlet other than music that would engage her and improve her mood. I wanted to find something better than a distraction that she could enjoy whilst remaining in her current memory loss identity, without having to push her back into the past with the use of music.

In session 1 and session 2, Participant 9 mentions that she used to enjoy reading. This extract is from the transcription of session 1:

Sam: *And how about books? Do you like reading?*
Participant 9: *I used to, but I don't read much now, no.*
Sam: *What kind of books did you used to like?*
Participant 9: *[She laughs] No, I can't think of anything.*
Sam: *That's OK.*
Participant 9: *I'm hopeless.*
Sam: *No, you're not at all. You're doing brilliantly. You say you used to read, but you don't read much now. Is there a reason for that, that you don't read now?*
Participant 9: *Hmm?*
Sam: *Is there a reason that you don't read much now?*
Participant 9: *No, no reason. No.*
Sam: *And can you think of any stories that you were told when you were growing up? Or any books from when you were little?*
Participant 9: *[She laughs] My memory just goes like that.*[31]

And she talks in more detail about a lost love of reading in session 2:

Sam: *How about books? Are there any books that you like?*
Participant 9: *[Still crying] I read [past tense] a lot but I don't remember any of them. My memory's terrible. My memory's completely gone, really.*

Sam: *Do you ever read now?*
Participant 9: *Yes, I do, but not very often.*
Sam: *And what kinds of things do you like to read?*
Participant 9: *Decent stories. Nothing much else.*
Sam: *Can you remember any stories that you were told when you were little? Or books that you read when you were little?*
Participant 9: *[Very sadly] My memory's just completely gone. I'm a hopeless person to talk to. You're not going to get any information from me at all. I'm hopeless.*
Sam: *I don't think you're hopeless at all.*[32]

In these two moments, Participant 9 shares that, although she used to enjoy reading, her memory loss means that she no longer feels that she can. Therefore, I decided that in the third session, I would experiment by sharing a quick fiction with her, which are entire stories in 300 words or less.[33] In doing this, my hope was that (a), Participant 9 would be able to remember some of the story by the time she reached the end, and (b), that she might enjoy the feeling of finishing a whole story. I began the session by sharing a short quick fiction that I had written, called, *Ready for Shakespeare*.[34] She read the fiction independently and then I asked her some questions about it. Despite being extremely tired during this session, the outcome was positive.

Sam: *Last time I spoke to you, we were talking about how you used to read a lot and that that was something that you really enjoyed. Do you think that if you had a set of really short stories, not just short stories, but really short stories like this... Do you think that's something that you might like to read and that that might be something that you would enjoy doing?*
Participant 9: *Yeah, possibly. Yeah, rather than very long things.*
Sam: *And, in terms of length, this is about 300 words long. Do you think that would be about the right length or do you think a little bit shorter would be better? Or a little bit longer?*
Participant 9: *No, that's not too long. No, that's about right.*
Sam: *You think that's about right?*
Participant 9: *Yes.*[35]

Here, Participant 9 comments that she finds the length of the story very manageable, and although the quick fiction is not to her taste, she believes that a story of around 300 words is something that she could enjoy reading. The recording of the session is enjoyable to listen to, and Participant 9 is in high spirits throughout, even though she is feeling very tired.

Sam: *...You said with a big book it feels a bit intimidating.*
Participant 9: *Yes.*

Sam: *So, do you think you would feel more inclined to have a go at reading something shorter?*
Participant 9: *Yes.*
Sam: *Well, good. Well, that's really fantastic. And having read it, can you remember anything about the story that you liked?*
Participant 9: *[Laughing] Not a lot, no! [Pause] I'm so tired.*
Sam: *That's OK. But you did you enjoy reading it at the time?*
Participant 9: *Yes, yes!*[36]

Interestingly, Participant 9 does not seem able to remember any specific details of the fiction, but she can remember how it made her feel, which is that it felt manageable, and although the story was not to her taste, she enjoyed reading it. In order to develop this idea further, and because she seemed to enjoy reading so much during session 3, I designed session 4 to involve reading and discussing three short pieces of writing.[37] I wanted her to read alongside me as a peer, rather than a teacher, to see if this would empower her. I chose to use a prose poem called, *Spring Day [Bath]* by Amy Lowell, a 100-word micro fiction called, *The Black Cat* by Jennifer Wilber, and a short-short story called, *Give It Up* by Franz Kafka.[38,39] Session 4 was by far the best session with Participant 9, who was calm and completely focused on all three texts, despite the fact that the lounge was particularly noisy that day. However, it did take a little while for her to feel confident enough to comment on the different texts. We began by reading *Spring Day*.

Sam: *OK, this is Participant number 9 session 4. So, we've just read together, Spring Day by Amy Lowell. Did you enjoy reading it?*
Participant 9: *Yes.*
Sam: *What did you like about it?*
Participant 9: *Nothing in particular.*
Sam: *Mmmhmm. Length-wise, was it about the right length, do you think?*
Participant 9: *Oh, yes.*[40]

At this point in the interview, Participant 9 seems a little nervous about sharing her thoughts on the text. However, she is completely engrossed in what she is reading and is able to ignore the unpleasant environmental noises around her. She re-reads the poem several times and it seems to calm her.

Sam: *And did you enjoy the feeling of getting to the end?*
Participant 9: *[Calmly] Yeah.*[41]

Although she does not make many comments on the poem, the length of the poem seems to suit her, and she becomes relaxed, which is unusual for Participant 9. The second piece of reading is her favourite of the three, as it triggers happy memories of some pets that she has owned during her life.

Sam: *I've got another one for you that's slightly different. This one's called The Black Cat. [Sam hands the micro fiction to Participant 9] It's slightly shorter. Have a read of it and see what you think of it, and I'll have a read of it as well.*

[Sam and Participant 9 sit next to each other and read their copies of The Black Cat. There is a lot of background noise in the lounge (television, teacups, coughing etc) but Participant 9 is completely focused on the reading. Participant 9 starts to laugh].

Sam: *I can see you're laughing. What are you... what about that tickled you?*
Participant 9: *[Laughing, she reads from the micro fiction] "I opened my door and let him in. He's now curled up in front of the fire. I don't think he will be leaving anytime soon, [she laughs] so I may as well get used to him." My cat was like that. [She laughs]*
Sam: *Did you have a cat?*
Participant 9: *I've had lots of cats.*
Sam: *Did you? So, reading this, did it remind you of what cats are like?*
Participant 9: *[Still looking at the text] Mmhmm.*[42]

Participant 9 is really happy at this moment in the session. The way that the cat is behaving in the microfiction is familiar to her, and the memory that it provokes of her cat is positive and makes her laugh. At this point, Participant 9 becomes more comfortable talking about the text.

Sam: *I think as well, it's quite a contrast to the last piece we just read. This is about warmth, isn't it? The cat's curled up in front of the fire, and obviously it's a different season. It's cold outside and the cat is doing that thing that cats do and they're a bit cheeky. They come in and they find the best spot in the house [Sam and Participant 9 laugh together] and then they don't want to go, do they?*
Participant 9: *No.*
Sam: *I think that obviously the writer doesn't... this black cat doesn't belong to her, but she sort of gives up and thinks, "Well, the cat's chosen me. It's chosen my fire. [It's chosen] my house and it doesn't want to go.*
Participant 9: *Yeah [she laughs].*
Sam: *What did you think of the fact that there were the two "Meows"?*
Participant 9: *Two meows?*
Sam: *Mm. So, it starts with a meow...*
Participant 9: *Oh yes. And then there's one here. [She points to the second "meow" in the text].*

Sam: *And then it ends with the meow.*
Participant 9: *Oh yeah.*
Sam: *What did you think of that?*
Participant 9: *[Laughing] It's like a cat, isn't it?*[43]

She is completely engrossed in the piece of writing by this point and is both happy and calm. She is really enjoying the session, and although I am still leading the conversation, she is able to talk to me as a peer. Now that she is feeling more confident, Participant 9 begins to share her ideas more willingly.

Sam: *Did you like that one?*
Participant 9: *Yeah.*
Sam: *Was there anything else that you liked about it or any words that particularly stood out?*
Participant 9: *It's funny. "I could use the company anyway" with a cat! [She laughs]*
Sam: *Mmhmm. And when she says "I could use the company anyway," what does that tell us about that person? The writer, or that character?*
Participant 9: *I think she's a bit lonely.*
Sam: *Yes. So, it makes you understand a bit about that character, doesn't it? And then the fact that the cat's come to stay with her feels like a nice thing...*
Participant 9: *Yes.*[44]

This ability to support her ideas with evidence from the text shows a level of sophistication to her critical thinking skills that she has not been able to demonstrate during our previous sessions. Although we are in conversation with one another she is thinking independently about the text and learning about it as she does so, which she is enjoying. The third text was the most challenging for Participant 9.

Sam: *...I've got one more for you to read, just one. [Sam hands the short-short story to Participant 9] It's the shortest. This is by a very famous author called, Kafka. Have a read of this one, it's a little bit different. This is called, Give It Up.*

[There is a pause as Sam and Participant 9 read the text. Again, there is a lot of background noise, but Participant 9 remains focused on the reading and does not become distracted].

Participant 9: *[Laughing] It's weird, this one!*
Sam: *[Laughing] You think this one is weird? So firstly, was there anything about it that stood out to you that you particularly enjoyed reading?*

Participant 9: *[Long pause whilst she takes a sip of her tea and reads the text carefully again] I'm not sure about this one!*
Sam: *[Laughing] How do you think the main character, or the person that is speaking is feeling?*
Participant 9: *[Another long pause. Participant 9 spends a long time pondering over the text.] It's a bit weird that! [She laughs].*[45]

Participant 9 finds this final text difficult to understand. However, she remains committed to the task and enjoys the challenge of trying to understand what might be happening in the story. As I realise that she is struggling to understand the text, I change the direction of the conversation and ask her what she thinks about the length of it.

Sam: *[Laughing] What did you think of the length of that one?*
Participant 9: *Hmm. I don't know.*
Sam: *That one's the shortest of the three, and it appears that that is the one that you like the least. I wonder if having a slightly longer one would suit you better?*
Participant 9: *It's weird!*[46]

For Participant 9, the word count of the text does not seem to have as big an impact as the content of the story. At this point, I try to end the session, but Participant 9 wants to continue to talk about the story.

Sam: *Well, thank you so much for taking the time to read those stories and to have a chat with me this morning. It's been really interesting to talk to you, as always. Is there anything else you want to say before I stop the recording about any of the things that you read this morning?*
Participant 9: *It's just, "Give it up! Give it up," he said, and turned away with a sudden jerk..." It's a weird, weird, thing!*
Sam: *Has it kept you... Has it made you think, "Ooh! Why is the policeman saying that?" Because there's a little element of mystery to that isn't there?*
Participant 9: *Yes, yeah.*
Sam: *Because we don't know why the policeman is laughing and saying, "Give it up! Give it up!" And the speaker or the character doesn't know either. So, we're sort of in the same position, aren't we?*
Participant 9: *[Enthusiastically] Yeah!*
Sam: *So, I guess that's where the mystery is, isn't it?*
Participant 9: *Yeah.*
Sam: *Wonderful. Well, thank you so much for talking to me. It's been lovely to speak to you.*
Participant 9: *[She laughs].*[47]

Participant 9 has so enjoyed this session. Reading together as peers has empowered her to be able to share her ideas about the texts with me, and there is something about reading the texts together that she seems to particularly enjoy. She has remained completely focused on all three of the texts throughout the session and has been calm and happy throughout. Not only has the session had a positive impact on Participant 9's mood, but she has demonstrated her ability to learn new things, despite her memory loss.

The fourth session with Participant 9 was a joy. She really enjoyed the reading that I gave to her, even when the final piece was not to her taste. After this session, I stayed to observe her for a little while, and she stayed in a peaceful and thoughtful state for the following half an hour, at which point I left the lounge to complete a session with another participant. When I left the nursing home that day (about an hour and a half later), I popped back into the lounge to see how Participant 9 was feeling. I found that she was crying, sitting next to a care worker who was attempting to distract her by trying to teach her how to make an origami swan, having just shown her a 'how-to' YouTube video on her small mobile phone. Participant 9 seemed to be very distressed by this. When I asked her if she was OK, the care worker answered, "She's fine." I then told the care worker that Participant 9 and I had been reading together that morning and she said, "Oh, she won't be able to do that. She can't read anymore." And at that, I left.

Case study 2

Participant 4: "It's not supposed to sound like that."

Participant 4 was another of the three ladies in the lounge. To look at, she was almost too tiny to be real. Her spine was curled into a perfect 'C' shape, and on the rare occasions that she did stand up she was only a little taller than my hip. Because of her rolled-up body, she would spend most of her time looking at the floor, presenting only the top of her head (which was covered by a neat, but balding grey bob) to the rest of the lounge. At moments when it was necessary to reveal her small and frowning face, her neck would click and bend itself backwards in a clumsy but robotic *ck ck ck*. When she spoke, her voice was hard and dusty as though she had an old coin stuck in her throat, and she constantly complained of feeling too cold. She proudly wore an air of a post-war mother, and, as such, she was passionate and cross in equal parts. There was a strong sense of pulse to the way in which she spat her repeated words, and as regularly as every three minutes, she would mutter the following song lyric like a spell; "If ever a devil was born, without a pair of horns, it was you."[48]

Of the three special chairs available in the lounge, Participant 4 had selected the chair on the right, which meant that Participant 8 sat between her and

Participant 9. This was not an accidental arrangement. Participant 9's confused sobs irritated Participant 4, and she would often be heard to angrily gurgle "Stop crying!" or "Shut up!" at the floor. Thankfully, Participant 8 was slightly more tolerant of Participant 9, and she was able to ease any potential conflict between the other two women from her central position by giggling and changing the subject to the topic of the day's weather. In contrast to the overbed tables that sat in front of Participant 9 and Participant 8, Participant 4's table was completely bare. This, I assumed, was because Participant 4 had insisted that her table was not to be decorated and was instead to be kept empty, aside from a small saucer of bourbon biscuits which she would nibble on throughout the day.

When we first met, and in spite of her appetite for conflict, Participant 4 and I got along well. Initially, she would ignore my attempts at small talk, but she would reach out and take my hand and cup it in both of hers, explaining that she was only doing so to "steal some heat." There was a queer feeling of common ground between us, and the penny dropped one afternoon when Participant 4 told me that she was a musician. She explained that, before the arthritis in her hands had set in, she had been a pianist. She also told me that her father had been a pianist and one of her sisters had been a violinist. The familiarity between our 55-years-apart childhoods laid the first stone for many interesting conversations about music, musical learning, and family, and I was hopeful that I might be able to use our sessions to help improve her low mood through some musical engagement.

Participant 4 completed four sessions with me. In our first session, she took part in a life story interview.[49] After this, I was keen to find out more about her musical background, so I wrote a personalised interview with a focus on her musical education.[50] In the third session, and because I was keen to learn more about the relationship that Participant 4 had with the song lyric that she recited so regularly, we listened to the song *Jezebel* together, and I asked her questions about how the song made her feel.[51,52] In our final session, I attempted to share a score with Participant 4 whilst we listened to a piece by Ludovico Einaudi.[53] However, as I will explain later, Participant 4 did not want to participate in that activity, so the session took a slightly different turn.

In her first session, Participant 4 is able to demonstrate that she has a relatively good long-term memory.[54]

Sam: *So, what is your earliest memory?*

Participant 4: *School. I don't know.*

Sam: *You don't know. OK, that's fine.*

Participant 4: *My earliest memory. I went to school. Remember my dad, my sisters. I had two sisters and they were both older than me. I was the baby. I know that my parents have gone and my two sisters are gone, but I've got a daughter.*[55]

This information about her family is easy for her to recall, and she goes on to share more information about her daughter.

Sam: *What's your daughter called?*
Participant 4: *****, **** and she was called ****...I chose it because she was three and a half pounds.*
Sam: *Aww.*
Participant 4: *But now she's huge! Bigger than me.*[56]

Her memory then becomes vaguer when asked about more general memories from the past.

Sam: *And can you remember any events from your childhood? Is there anything that stands out to you?*
Participant 4: *Not really. Nothing special. I went to school. Mr ****** was our headmaster. I don't know.*
Sam: *And how about your teenage years? Between the ages of thirteen and nineteen. Is there anything that stands out to you from those years?*
Participant 4: *Boyfriends. I don't know.*
Sam: *And how about your adult years? Are there any events that stand out as being particularly significant?*
Participant 4: *Not that I remember.*[57]

At this point, I return to questions about her family, which she is able to answer.

Sam: *And you mentioned your family. So, you said you were the youngest of three?*
Participant 4: *What?*
Sam: *You said you're the youngest of three daughters. Is that right?*
Participant 4: *Yes.*
Sam: *And then did you marry?*
Participant 4: *I did. He's dead and gone.*
Sam: *What was his name?*
Participant 4: ******.*
Sam: *What was he like?*
Participant 4: *My world. He's been dead for about a couple of years I suppose, but he was all the world to me. [Fiddles with the wedding band and engagement ring on her wedding finger].*[58]

At this point, Participant 4's mood changes. She obviously feels a great deal of sadness when talking about her husband's death, and she takes a moment to reflect as she fiddles with the rings on her hands. I then ask her to tell me a little more about her daughter.

Sam: *And you have a daughter, you said?*
Participant 4: *A daughter, ****. And she was called **** because she was so small. There we are.*
Sam: *And does **** have any children?*
Participant 4: *What?*
Sam: *Does **** have any children? Do you have grandchildren?*
Participant 4: *No. She's not married. She goes to work.*
Sam: *What does she do? What's her job?*
Participant 4: *Works at ******.*[59]

Participant 4 has forgotten that she has already shared the anecdote of the reason for her daughter's name. There is a strange sense of disconnect between Participant 4 and her daughter (her only living close relative) at this point in the conversation, and, whilst Participant 4 does not seem to feel sad that she does not have grandchildren, she does seem to blame this on the fact that her daughter has not married and has worked 'instead'. There is a feeling at this moment in the interview that the differences between Participant 4 and her daughter are not simply generational, and that she finds it difficult to relate to the choices that her daughter has made. This, I assume, is because the choices that her daughter has made about family are so different to her own. She then goes on to talk in more detail about her father.

Sam: *And can you think of someone who's been a really positive influence in your life?*
Participant 4: *My father, I suppose. You did as he told you. I don't know.*
Sam: *What was your father like?*
Participant 4: *World. ******** ******. [She shares his full name]*[60]

Here, Participant 4 explains how important her father was to her by describing him, as she did her husband, as being her "*world.*" She hints that her father was a figure of authority by saying, "*You did as he told you.*" but this appears to be a positive memory for her. This, alongside the fact that she has already shared the memory of her former (male) head teacher's name, is interesting, particularly when she has yet to mention her mother at all during the interview. I then began to question Participant 4 on memories from a more recent past, which she finds harder to answer.

Sam: *These next questions are about things that you like, about your personal taste. Can you think of a television programme that you've particularly enjoyed over the years?*
Participant 4: *I...no. If something's on, I think, 'Oh, is that on? I'll watch that', but that's how far it goes.*

Sam: *And how about a film? Do you have a favourite film?*
Participant 4: *No.*
Sam: *And how about books? Do you like to read?*
Participant 4: *Not now. Not now.*
Sam: *Are there any books that you can remember...*
Participant 4: *I can't.*
Sam: *OK, that's fine.*
Participant 4: *You what?*
Sam: *That's fine. And how about stories you were told when you were little? Are there any stories that you can remember from when you were growing up?*
Participant 4: *I don't think we had stories when we were growing up because father went to work and mother didn't have time.*[61]

Participant 4 is demonstrating that she has trouble with her short-term memory, but she is also admitting that she does not enjoy engaging in any activities for entertainment purposes. The first mention of her mother is also interesting, and what I can infer from "*father went to work and mother didn't have time*" is that her mother stayed at home to look after Participant 4 and her two sisters, but she was so busy looking after the home that she did not have time to read her three daughters a story. There is a tension that exists between the working mother and the stay-at-home mother for Participant 4. Whilst she seems to disapprove of her daughter's choice not to marry and have children, she also seems to favour her father over her mother, even though her mother married and had children, which is something that she seems to value. At this point in the interview, I assume that Participant 4 has also been a stay-at-home mother to her daughter, ****. Next, Participant 4 shares some details about her musical upbringing.

Sam: *And do you have a favourite song or piece of music that you particularly like?*
Participant 4: *I used to like music that I played, but I can't play...can't do it anymore. And I don't remember, no.*
Sam: *What did you used to play?*
Participant 4: *Piano.*
Sam: *Can you remember any pieces of music that you liked playing on the piano?*
Participant 4: *No.*
Sam: *But did you enjoy playing the piano?*
Participant 4: *I don't know. I played...I had to play the piano first. I had to. But I can't do it now. My fingers get too stiff.*[62]

Participant 4 not only tells me that she used to play the piano (which she had already told me many times during our informal conversations in the lounge) but she also shares that she, "*had to play the piano first,*" suggesting that (a), she did not have a choice whether to learn to play the piano or not, and that (b), she perhaps learned another instrument that she has not mentioned. Also, as I already know that her father was a musician, my understanding is that it was her father who insisted that she learned to play it. At this point in the interview, I change the subject to the topic of religion.

Sam: *Do you have a religion?*
Participant 4: *I used to...Church of England. I used to be in the choir. I used to ring the bells. What else did we used to do? What else do you do in Church?*
Sam: *Ooh, I'm not sure. I mean, there are lots of jobs you can do in a church, aren't there? People do things with the flowers and all kinds of things, don't they? The readings or teas and coffees afterwards or...people do all kinds of things for a church, don't they?*
Participant 4: *Well, I did it because I was told to.*
Sam: *Can you remember any of the songs you used to sing in the choir?*
Participant 4: *Hymns. No songs. Hymns.*[63]

This conversation about religious beliefs seems to trigger more memories about the musical activities that Participant 4 engaged with during her upbringing which, once again, she says she did because she was, "*told to,*" presumably by her father. It also suggests that, to her, her relationship with religion is linked to her relationship with her family. Participant 4 then answers the following question very quickly, without pausing to think:

Sam: *Good. And this is a bit of a tricky question, but if you look back over your life and try to imagine it as a story, what do you think the main message or theme of that story would be?*
Participant 4: *Do as your mother said.*[64]

These words are interesting as Participant 4's mother has been a largely absent voice during the rest of the interview, and this extremely direct answer to a fairly complex question suggests that it may have been Participant 4's mother that was the authoritarian figure in her life, rather than her father. The end of the interview surprised me even more.

Sam: *Fantastic... That's the end of my questions, but is there anything else you'd like to tell me? Interesting things that happened in your life or jobs that you've had?*
Participant 4: *I only had one job.*
Sam: *What was your job?*
Participant 4: *Erm, nursing.*

Sam: *And did you work locally? Did you work in ******** **** as a nurse?*

Participant 4: *I worked, yes. I worked locally. I think I might have worked down in Cornwall, but I worked here locally.*

Sam: *And did you enjoy nursing?*

Participant 4: *I think so. I kept at it. You were a nurse and that was it. Looked after the patients.*

Sam: *Fantastic. Well, thank you so much for talking to me today. I'll stop that there. [Turns off the dictaphone].*[65]

It is a shock to learn that Participant 4 has had a career as a nurse at this point in the interview. She seems so conflicted between working and not working and mothering and not mothering, and although she claims to like being told what to do, it is unclear whether the main figure or authority in her life has been her father or her mother.

During the time that I spent in the company of Participant 4, our relationship became increasingly complicated. Initially, we had got along very well. Her direct nature had made me laugh (which she seemed to enjoy, although she would never laugh along with me) and in many ways, she reminded me of my own grandmother. When I would enter the lounge, she would always be frighteningly still, and curved over in her perfect 'C' shape, as if in a very deep sleep. However, after a while, the familiar sound of my voice seemed to animate her, and her neck would perform its reverse clack and click so that she could show her face to me. I never saw her smile, but there was a softness to her face in those brief moments, and she would offer a semi-friendly "hello." Then, although her body would stay completely still, her owl eyes would follow me keenly as I moved around the lounge, and in those moments, I began to feel on my skin that she liked me and hated me all at once. The strange tension that this created would only be released when I eventually sat beside her, at which point she would take my hand to "steal some heat" (she took to inspecting them before she cupped them, palms up, then palms down) and there would then be a cooling down period as she allowed herself to breathe more deeply, before curling back into the animal comfort of her perfect 'C'.

This mysterious reaction from Participant 4 puzzled me for some time. To begin with, she seemed to enjoy the conversations that we had, particularly when we spoke about music. I inferred from the performance repertoire that we discussed that she had been a competent musician, and we talked many times about musical memories from our upbringings. One morning, she described in detail to me how the butterflies in her tummy had felt during a first public performance in a large church hall, and in return, I told her how my fledgling heart had been broken during a piano recital at the age of nine when I lost my place in the music and had to stop. She told me about friendly family arguments about performance techniques during cold big-coat walks on the beach, and I told her how my sister (a violinist) and I had played Christmas Carols to my grandparents every Christmas morning. However, even though we had shared these cherished memories with one another, a strong underlying feeling of tension developed between us, and it was not until I observed her whilst playing a short recital to all of the residents in the lounge that I realised why.

I had offered to play some flute recitals to the residents during my time at the nursing home as a thank you for allowing me to carry out my fieldwork there. These sessions varied greatly (one of particular note is explained in Case Study 4) and ranged from performing a 45-minute recital in one lady's room at 10 am (whilst she drank a can of Fosters that she took from the crate underneath her bed), to performances to larger groups in the lounge and other communal spaces.

I first played to the group in the lounge on a Friday morning after I had been visiting the home for about two weeks. I positioned myself in front of the large television, which had been ceremoniously muted for the occasion. A larger group than usual had gathered, which included several residents who were non-verbal wheelchair users, some care workers, and some relatives who happened to be visiting. Participant 4 was in her usual seat (as were Participant 8 and Participant 9) and a care worker (who had pulled up another, harder chair on the other side of Participant 4) was holding her hand. I was particularly looking forward to playing for Participant 4 and had planned a repertoire with her in mind. Before the performance, she was curled over in her usual 'C' shape and was facing the floor.

When I started to play my first piece, the care worker who was sitting next to Participant 4 enthusiastically said, "Come on, *********, lift your head up! You'll enjoy this!". However, Participant 4 continued to face the floor for the duration of the first three pieces, and she was so still that I assumed that she was asleep. However, whilst playing my fourth piece, I began to hear a familiar grumbling noise coming from Participant 4, and I wondered whether she was about to tell Participant 9 to stop crying, as she always did. The grumbling got louder and louder, and then I heard the care worker who was holding her hand say, "You *do* like this! Don't be rude! It takes a lot of years to be able to play like that!" When I had finished playing the fourth piece, I heard that Participant 4 was in fact saying, "It's not supposed to sound like that!" over and over again. She looked visibly distressed and refused to lift her head throughout the rest of the performance. When I had finished and was packing away, she was still repeatedly saying, "It's not supposed to sound like that" and after that Friday morning, our relationship sadly became progressively problematic.

The transcription of session 2 with Participant 4 is indicative of the discussions that I would have with her in the lounge after that first performance.[66] She would begin by being quite amiable, but as soon as I mentioned music, she would try to end the conversation. An informal conversation with a care worker revealed that Participant 4 had been repeating "It's not supposed to sound like that" on a loop ever since the concert, so I decided that I would not play any music to her during our second session, and chose instead to ask her a series of questions about her musical upbringing, which she seemed to like discussing. The session took place in the lounge and Participant 9 was loudly sobbing two chairs down throughout. At the beginning of the interview, Participant 4 tells me some information that she has told me many times before.

Sam: *So, *********, have you ever played an instrument?*
Participant 4: *Piano.*
Sam: *You played the piano. And did you enjoy playing the piano?*
Participant 4: *Did I ever what?*
Sam: *Did you enjoy playing the piano?*
Participant 4: *[Enthusiastically] Oh yes, when I played it. My father taught me.*
Sam: *And could your father play the piano as well then?*
Participant 4: *Yes.*[67]

At this point, Participant 4 seems to have (a) forgotten that she has told me this many times and (b) forgotten that she does not like talking to me about this anymore. I then probe a little further, to see if she will share any new information with me whilst she is feeling in a positive mood.

Sam: *And what kind of music did you play?*
Participant 4: *God, I don't know. Classical.*
Sam: *Classical music. And have you ever seen any live music? Did you ever go and watch any concerts?*
Participant 4: *We couldn't afford it.*
Sam: *And do you enjoy listening to music now?*
Participant 4: *Not particularly.*[68]

Here, it is as though Participant 4 has remembered that she no longer likes talking to me about music, but she does not seem to know why. She also reveals some financial hardship from her childhood. The environment in the lounge then becomes extremely noisy.

Sam: *Why don't you like listening to music?*
Participant 4: *Didn't know, I don't like. [Participant 4 looks deep in thought, as if she is thinking of more that she would like to say. The lounge is extremely noisy now. Some care workers are trying to distract Participant 9 in order to calm her down. There is a long pause]. Bloody noise.*
Sam: *Do you find the noise distracting?*
Participant 4: *Couldn't care less. I can grumble, can't I?*
Sam: *So, do you not enjoy listening to music now?*
Participant 4: *No.*
Sam: *Why is that?*
Participant 4: *What, looking at, listening to that noise? [Angrily, and as though she is quoting someone else] What are you looking at that noise for?*[69]

The intriguing thing at this point of the interview is the apparent blurring of Participant 4's senses. She seems to be confusing hearing and seeing. This might be because she sees images when she hears music, and the change in delivery with "What are you looking at that noise for?" introduces a third voice into our conversation, suggesting that they are words that are not necessarily her own. I then try to understand how listening to music makes Participant 4 feel.

Sam: *When you were younger, did you used to like listening to music?*
Participant 4: *I never went out of my way to play...to listen to music.*
Sam: *OK. Was there ever...*
Participant 4: *What?*
Sam: *Was there ever a kind of music or a piece of music that made you feel happy when you listened to it?*
Participant 4: *No. Not that I remember.*
Sam: *And, have there ever been any pieces of music that have made you feel sad when you've listened to them?*
Participant 4: *No. I don't know. I don't know.*[70]

Participant 4 is feeling cross at this moment in our conversation. She is insistent that she gets no enjoyment from listening to music and she wants me to stop asking her questions about it, so her answers are brief and dismissive. I then try to find out the connection that Participant 4 has to the song lyric that she recites regularly.

Sam: *Can you remember any lyrics to any songs?*
Participant 4: *Play the music and I might.*
Sam: *OK, so if I played you a song, do you think you might be able to remember some of the words?*
Participant 4: *I might but it depends on the music... on the song. If ever the devil was born, without a pair of horns, it was you.*
Sam: *Is that a song lyric?*
Participant 4: *What dear?*
Sam: *Is that a song lyric?*
Participant 4: *That was what?*
Sam: *Those words you just said, what was that? If ever the...*
Participant 4: *[She half-sings] If ever the devil was born, without a pair of horns, it was you.*
Sam: *And is that a song?*
Participant 4: *It is.*
Sam: *Do you know who it's by?*
Participant 4: *I haven't the foggiest. Used to be, I think...You heard it on the radio, I think. I don't remember. [Half-singing] I don't remember. I don't remember the 5th of November, gunpowder treason and plot. I see no reason why gunpowder and treason should ever be forgot.*[71]

By now, Participant 4 is tired of the session and is feeling frustrated with me. She no longer wishes to speak to me, and she starts to pretend that she cannot hear me, hoping that I will end the conversation. However, when she remembers the song lyric, "If ever the devil was born, without a pair of horns, it was you," she is impelled to say it, and she even half-sings it. Then, when she says, "I don't remember," this triggers a memory of another song, which she also half-sings. I then try to find out a little about Participant 4's relationship with music and memory.

Sam:	*Are there any pieces of music that bring back memories for you?*
Participant 4:	*[Quickly] No.*
Sam:	*Are there any pieces of music that remind you of a time in your life?*
Participant 4:	*No. Too long ago. Too long ago.*[72]

Participant 4 is adamant that there are no pieces of music that bring back memories for her. The interview ends with me trying to find out if there is some music that Participant 4 would like to listen to.

Sam:	*And if a musician or somebody who could play an instrument came in here and played to you, would you enjoy that?*
Participant 4:	*It all depends how good they are.*
Sam:	*And are there any instruments that you like listening to being played?*
Participant 4:	*No.*
Sam:	*Well, thank you so much for talking to me today. I really appreciate your time.*[73]

This insistence that there are no instruments that she would like to listen to is the saddest moment of the session. This, combined with the distress that Participant 4 seemed to feel during my first group performance in the lounge and her confusion between hearing and seeing music, suggests that there is something more at play when it comes to Participant 4's relationship with music, which seems to have changed drastically since her childhood.

When I was planning the third session for Participant 4, I decided that I wanted to investigate her relationship with the song lyric that she recited so often so I wrote an interview that started with us listening to the song together.[74] I was apprehensive about playing some music to Participant 4, and I knew that her reaction was likely to be negative. At the beginning of the interview, Participant 4 immediately recognises the song that is playing.

Sam: *OK, this is Participant 4, session 3. We are going to start by listening to a piece of music.*

[Sam starts playing Jezebel by Frankie Lane].[75]

Participant 4: *[Singing along to the music] If ever a devil was born, without a pair of horns, it was you. [Then speaking] Jezebel.*[76]

When Participant 4 hears the familiar lyrics, she sings along, which then triggers the memory of the name of the song. At this moment, she is surprisingly happy to hear the song and she sings along to some of the other lyrics that she recognises as it plays. However, when the song stops, and my questions about music begin, Participant 4 becomes deliberately standoffish.

Sam: *OK, I noticed you were singing along to some of that. Do you remember it?*
Participant 4: *What?*
Sam: *Do you remember the song?*
Participant 4: *What song?*
Sam: *The song we just listened to.*
Participant 4: *The song we what?*
Sam: *The song we were just listening to there. Do you remember the song?*
Participant 4: *[Pause] Jezebel.*
Sam: *Mmmhmm. And can you remember any more of the lyrics than the ones that you were singing along to?*
Participant 4: *[Angrily] I don't know what the song is.*
Sam: *We were just listening to Jezebel by Frankie Lane.*
Participant 4: *[Long pause] I'm useless dear.*[77]

It is unclear whether Participant 4 has forgotten the song that she has just listened to, or if she is pretending to have forgotten it, in an attempt to stop me asking her questions about it. I suspect that, seeing as she is able to remember the name of the song in this short passage, she is pretending to have forgotten it. She continues to be disobliging as the interview continues.

Sam: *Do you remember hearing the song before? Yes? And, does it remind you of anything when you listen to it?*
Participant 4: *No.*
Sam: *No? OK. And how does it make you feel when you listen to it?*
Participant 4: *Nothing.*
Sam: *Nothing. OK. And can you remember how old you were when you first heard it?*
Participant 4: *Five hundred and fifty-eight, I suppose.*
Sam: *Five hundred and fifty-eight. And, are there any other songs that you can remember the lyrics to?*
Participant 4: *I don't think so.*[78]

The breakdown of the relationship between myself and Participant 4 is having a negative impact on the interview by this point, and my feeling is that she is being deliberately obtuse when she says that she first heard the song when she was "Five hundred and fifty-eight" years old. I now begin to attempt to bring the interview to a conclusion, but am surprised by Participant 4's answer to my next question.

Sam: *And, can you think of any other lyrics that you can remember now?*

Participant 4: *Yes, it comes along with the song.*

Sam: *And do you have a favourite song?*

Participant 4: *No.*

Sam: *Did you enjoy listening to that today?*

Participant 4: *What?*

Sam: *Did you enjoy listening to Jezebel today?*

Participant 4: *Did I enjoy listening to something?*

Sam: *Yes, today.*

Participant 4: *[Long pause] Yes, I think so.*[79]

Whilst Participant 4 is adamant that she does not want to talk about how the song makes her feel, she does admit that she enjoyed listening to it. It feels as though she is being honest here, and whilst she cannot necessarily remember listening to the song at the beginning of the interview by this point, she does remember that she enjoyed the feeling of listening to it. As the mood seems to have shifted, I attempt to continue the interview.

Sam: *And, does the song make you think of anything at all? Does it remind you of anything?*

Participant 4: *Cold. [Suddenly much louder] Cold coming in!*

[The hairdresser who is visiting responds to Participant 4 by saying, "I'll shut that door, *********. ****** *[Participant 8] was hot.]*

Sam: *OK. Well, thank you so much for talking to me. It's been lovely to talk to you, as always.*

Participant 4: *[I'm] useless to you.*[80]

This is a sad ending to this interview, in which I have struggled to communicate with Participant 4. She dislikes talking to me about music, but she is not able to articulate the reason why, as she may not know the reason herself. Her final, "[I'm] useless to you." is a big shift in tone from the rest of the interview, and it comes with a sense of apology.

After our difficult third session, I waited a while until I approached Participant 4 to ask if she was willing to have a fourth. During this period, she continued to react to my arrival in the lounge with her strange know you/do not know you, like you/hate you glare. However, she seemed to warm to me again, and she was very happy to talk to me and "steal some heat" (palms up, palms down) if I did not mention music. This time allowed me to reflect on our previous three sessions, and I wondered if listening to some music whilst reading the score might help to support the aural/visual nature of Participant 4's musical skills, so I tentatively planned a session in which I hoped to play her some music and read the score with her at the same time.

Unfortunately, Participant 4 was adamant that she did not want to take part in the task that I had planned for her fourth session. She was horrified when I showed her the piece of music and insisted that she did not want to look at it, nor did she want to listen to it. However, her brief scan of the score seemed to trigger some memories about her childhood piano lessons, and she soon calmed down as she began to tell me about her piano teacher. At this point, I asked her if she was happy for me to record the conversation, and she confirmed that she was. She begins by confirming the name of her piano teacher.[81]

Sam:	*OK, this is Participant 4, session 4. So, you were telling me about your piano teacher just then. What was your piano teacher's name?*
Participant 4:	*Mrs **********.*
Sam:	*And what was she like?*
Participant 4:	*Well, I was only about 10.*
Sam:	*And did you like going to your piano lessons?*
Participant 4:	*What?*
Sam:	*Did you like going to your piano lessons?*
Participant 4:	*I don't know. I didn't know. I went because I had to. I went to the shops to do the shopping. I went to Mrs ********** because I had to. [Unrecognisable speech].*[82]

Once again, Participant 4 reveals that she went to her piano lessons because she "had to," although it is not clear who it was that made her go. Her memory for names of people in a position of authority during her childhood is impressive, and I am reminded here of her ability to easily recall the name of her school head teacher during our first session. Next, Participant 4 is able to remember how often she played the piano as a child.

Sam:	*And did you do your piano practice? Did you practice at home?*
Participant 4:	*Yes.*
Sam:	*Did you have a piano at home to practice on between your lessons?*
Participant 4:	*Yes.*
Sam:	*And how many lessons did you say you had a week?*
Participant 4:	*Lessons?*
Sam:	*How often did you visit your piano teacher?*
Participant 4:	*I had to go and play the piano every evening. I don't know how often she was there. I would have been there during the day, doing something. She didn't come in the evenings.*[83]

Participant 4 is able to remember an impressive amount of information about the regularity of her childhood music practice. She also reiterates that she, "had to go and play the piano every evening" suggesting that her musical education was not her choice. However, she still does not reveal who it was that made her learn to play the piano. I then asked her a question about performances, to which I already know the answer from our informal conversations in the lounge.

Sam: *And did you ever do any performances playing the piano? Did you ever play to an audience?*
Participant 4: *I did actually.*
Sam: *Did you?*
Participant 4: *Mrs **********'s concerts.*
Sam: *So did she used to...*
Participant 4: *What?*
Sam: *Did...was it Mrs ********** you said?*
Participant 4: *Yes.*
Sam: *Did she used to have concerts for all her pupils to play in?*
Participant 4: *She had concerts for people to go and sit and listen. And it was at... [pause] either the gas office or wherever, and [pause] I forget where it was.*[84]

Whilst Participant 4 has been reluctant to provide information about her engagement with music in sessions 2 and 3, she is very keen to talk about it here and spends a long time trying to remember the name of the venue in which the concerts took place. She then seems to remember that she does not like to talk to me about music, and her answers suddenly become dismissive.

Sam: *And can you remember any of the pieces that you learned to play?*
Participant 4: *No. 1000 times no.*
Sam: *And in those concerts in the in the gas office with Mrs **********'s pupils, do you remember how it felt to play to an audience?*
Participant 4: *She used to... let's give it a concert every year or something. [Long pause] I'm old. Old.*[85]

Her "1000 times no" is delivered with irritation and at this point in the conversation I begin to worry that she no longer wishes to speak to me, as has happened in the previous two sessions. During her long pause, she seems to be trying to remember something, but then she gives up, saying, "I'm old. Old" in apology. I then ask her some further questions to which I already know the answer, and Participant 4's answers continue to be dismissive.

Sam: *Did you enjoy playing in those concerts? Did you enjoy playing to an audience?*

Participant 4: *No. Very nervous.*
Sam: *You got very nervous. Can you remember what that feeling felt like? Being nervous?*
Participant 4: *[Shakes head].*
Sam: *And were your family invited to come and watch you play?*
Participant 4: *I don't know. I expect so.*
Sam: *And how long ago did you last play the piano?*
Participant 4: *I don't know.*
Sam: *Did you have a piano in your house when you were an adult?*
Participant 4: *[Nods] I did.*[86]

It feels as though Participant 4 has given up on the conversation now. However, the opportunity to speak about her father reanimates her.

Sam: *So in your family, when you were a child, did you say that you and your sister learned to play and your dad...*
Participant 4: *My elder sister did, but my other one didn't. She played the violin.*
Sam: *Ah, OK. Did you like the violin?*
Participant 4: *Eh?*
Sam: *Did you like the sound of the violin?*
Participant 4: *My father played violin.*
Sam: *Oh, he played the violin as well? And was that your dad's job? Was he a musician?*
Participant 4: *No.*[87]

Participant 4 so enjoys talking about her father that she uses my question about the sound of the violin to share that her father played the violin as well as the piano, which is information that she had not revealed to me beforehand during our many conversations about music. I ended the conversation by asking Participant 4 if she has any other memories of her time as a pianist that she would like to tell me.

Sam: *And do you have any other memories that stick out in your mind about being a pianist, or of playing the piano? Or are there any pieces that you can remember playing, or anything that you enjoyed doing?*
Participant 4: *I don't remember. [Half-singing] I remember, I remember, the 5th of November.*
Sam: *Well, it's been lovely to talk to you. Thank you so much for talking to me this morning. Thank you.*
Participant 4: *I'm very tired. Sorry I'm not very...*
Sam: *No, it's been lovely to talk to you. Thank you.*[88]

The apology at the end of the session does not feel like it is offered to me, and I wonder why Participant 4 seems to apologise in a variety of ways throughout all four of our sessions. But the most curious thing about the end of the interview is the resurgence of the song lyric, "I remember, I remember, the 5th of November," which she also said in session 2. However, in session 2, what she actually said was, "I don't remember. I don't remember the 5th of November, gunpowder treason and plot. I see no reason why gunpowder and treason should ever be forgot."[89]

I was disappointed when my time with Participant 4 came to an end, as I had been hopeful that I would be able to find a way to lift her mood by engaging her in some musical activities. Unfortunately, the change in hearing that memory loss brings was too distressing for Participant 4, and even clouded her boundaries between hearing and seeing at times. This meant that, sadly, Participant 4 was happiest when the music, which had been a large part of her life, was turned off. However, the loudest silence in my sessions with Participant 4 was her almost invisible mother. I am left to question who she was, where she is, and why, when asked what the message or theme of the story of her life would be, Participant 4 answered, "Do as you mother said."[90]

Case study 3

Participant 3: "I am fifteen years old."

Have you ever had a conversation with someone that was asleep? That is how it felt to talk to Participant 3. Her voice sounded like a secret and had the same ethereal timbre that is produced when a violinist dreams up the harmonics that hide inside their strings. This hypnogogic-harmonic storytelling style made me feel as though Participant 3 was letting me listen to the many things that were lingering and unfolding inside the shell of each of her precious words, and my sessions with her gave me an insight into the time-travelling world of the memory loss experience.

Participant 3 never came to the lounge, so I would visit her in her room, where I would find her sitting in an armchair that stood with its back to the window. The room was impeccably tidy and looked eerily identical on each of my four visits. Because of this, entering the room became cumulatively stranger over the weeks, and when I arrived for the final session, I felt like I was walking behind a glass screen of a scene in a museum, with Participant 3 playing the part of the mannequin, and me being the lost child. The blue walls were barely visible beneath a myriad of framed black and white photographs of very young babies. The baby/ies in the photographs were all sleeping and were so young that it was impossible to tell whether they were photographs of one or multiple children. On the bed sat a large, life-like stuffed ginger cat that was also sleeping, and several strings of rosary beads hung precariously but uniformly from the corner of the bedside table. Thick net curtains blocked the view of the street outside, but the stubborn light of the sun illuminated Participant 3 in her spot by the window, and on occasions when a bus would drive past, the room would be dipped into a flash of momentary darkness, only to blink back to life and light seconds later.

Each time I met her, I would find Participant 3 sitting in her armchair in a contented, dreamlike state. She would be in exactly the same position, with her small feet (which were always wearing the same pair of fluffy Christmas socks) stretched out in front of her, and her hands tucked politely on her lap. She was a petite but healthy-looking woman with wide and glossy kingfisher-blue eyes and a head of neat, curly grey hair. The television (which had to be operated by a plug that she could not reach) would always be playing when I arrived, but she gave it no attention, choosing instead to sit peacefully with her thoughts. Despite her apparent happiness to exist inside her private world, Participant 3 did not mind being interrupted, and always seemed to be pleased with the promise of some company when I arrived. She would greet me by complimenting my outfit ("Those are lovely flowers on your dress.") before asking me if I knew how to turn off the television, and once the plug was off, we would begin to talk.

Participant 3 completed four sessions with me. Like all primary participants, she completed a life story interview during her first session.[91] During that session, I was interested in the way in which she dreamily responded to certain words in a style of free association, so in the second session I planned a free association word task.[92] In our third session, having learned that Participant 3 had grown up on a farm, I played her some environmental farm sounds to see if this would trigger any memories from her childhood.[93] In the final session, I showed her some images of some of the things that she had had on her farm (chickens, cows, sheep, and hay bales) so that I could compare the way in which sound and vision might trigger memories for Participant 3 in different or similar ways.[94]

In her first session, Participant 3 is very keen to talk about her life, and although she finds some specific details hard to remember, she uses the memories that she has available to her to speak enthusiastically about her family and her upbringing.[95]

Participant 3: *I worked hard all my life.*

Sam: *So, this is Participant number 3. And I just wanted to ask you, my first question is; what's your earliest memory?*

Participant 3: *Ah, well, we were a big family. Little ones coming along lovely. Very exciting. And then they all grew up. But I've got two lovely brothers. Three lovely brothers at home. And we all stay good friends. Which is nice.*

Sam: *That's lovely. Can you describe an event from your childhood that stands out as being something that was really important?*

Participant 3: *I was too busy to take any notice. We had cows, sheep, and all that kind of thing. So I was always running in hens and chickens. Running in and out and shopping.*[96]

Participant 3 begins our conversation by mentioning the farm that she grew up on, and the fact that she was always busy. She also mentions that she has a large family, although specific details are missing at this point. She then shares a more vivid memory, when asked about memories from her adult years.

Sam: *And how about your adult life? So, anywhere from being sort of twenty to now, is there anything, any events in your life that are really, really significant?*

Participant 3: *I lost my brother, big brother, and that will always be there. His name was *******. He was six foot tall and away at work. So he came home and I always remember him coming up the little road to our house and settling down. He was a lovely young man. And then he got that thing in his legs. People dying with it. And eventually it killed him. When he was sitting there, quiet man. So there. That's the end. So many people were lost because there was nobody there to see them.*

Sam: *How old was ******* when he passed away?*

Participant 3: *Sorry?*

Sam: *How old was ******* when he passed away?*

Participant 3: *Twenty-four, I think.*

Sam: *Right.*

Participant 3: *He was still growing. He was very tall. You'd have to look up at him. But he was a nice chap, a good man.*[97]

Participant 3 remembers many specific details about the death of her older brother, and she seems to be pleased to be able to tell me about him. She is very open about the pain that his death has caused her ("I lost my brother, big brother, and that will always be there.") and as the interview progresses, it is clear that this is the most detailed memory that she holds from her past. Participant 3 then begins to talk about her children.

Sam: *And did you have children?*

Participant 3: *Oh, we had lots of children in those days. Everybody had children.*

Sam: *How many children did you have?*

Participant 3: *There were nine of us. Kids. Most of them are still at home. Working from home.*

Sam: *And how about grandchildren? Do you have grandchildren?*

Participant 3: *Did I have what?*

Sam: *Grandchildren.*

Participant 3: *Oh, I've got loads of those. I count them on my fingers. I've got four at home and three still at school. I was always wondering after children. But they were good. Good kids.*

Sam: *And did you like spending time with children?*

Participant 3: *Oh, I did. I loved it. I still do.*[98]

Participant 3 is from a very large family and has had many children and grandchildren, which she has enjoyed. However, she is confused about whether she is telling me about her siblings, her children, or her grandchildren. Then, when asked questions that she finds it harder to answer, she continues to talk about the work ethic of her farming family and the way in which they lived as children.

Sam:	*And who would you say has had a really positive influence on your life? If you were to pick one person, is there anybody that really stands out as having a really positive influence?*
Participant 3:	*Everybody worked so hard.*
Sam:	*So is that something that's important to you?*
Participant 3:	*It was good. We were always together.*
Sam:	*And is there anybody that you can think of that has had a negative impact on your life?*
Participant 3:	*Not really.*[99]

The theme of working hard and not having enough time then becomes more prevalent as the interview progresses.

Sam:	*The next questions are more about your personal sense of taste and the things that you like. So, can you think of a television programme that you've particularly enjoyed or a series that you've particularly liked?*
Participant 3:	*When the young ones were growing up, they were choosing this, so we would always watch the programmes that everybody liked. But I never had enough time.*
Sam:	*How about a film? Is there a film that you particularly like?*
Participant 3:	*I used to like that one. That game on television.*
Sam:	*Can you remember what it was called?*
Participant 3:	*No.*
Sam:	*And how about books? Do you like to read?*
Participant 3:	*I haven't got time for books. I used to read to the children but… I still read with them, but the young ones are growing up now.*
Sam:	*Can you think back to any stories that you were told, or that you read when you were little?*
Participant 3:	*Oh, we never had enough time. We were always busy. We had lambs, sheep, and cows and chickens. You name it, we had it. So I was always running after something or other. But I enjoyed it. We had a good childhood. We had a long way to go to school.*[100]

At this moment, Participant 3 has become very confused about which period of her life she is talking about. When she says, "I haven't got time for books. I used to read to the children but… I still read with them, but the young ones are growing up now." it is unclear whether she is talking about her children, or her grandchildren, or both. And when, in the next breath, she says, "We had a good childhood. We had a long way to go to school" she is then talking about her own childhood once more. Participant 3 then shares a little about the role that music has had in her life.

Sam: *Do you have a favourite song or piece of music?*

Participant 3: *Oh, we had, my mother played the accordion very well. She still does. We all enjoyed the music and the dancing. But the trouble was we grew up so quickly. There was always a little one to worry about.*

Sam: *And can you remember any of the songs or the pieces of music that your mother used to play?*

Participant 3: *[Long pause] We had a very happy childhood.*[101]

Participant 3's concerns about how quickly time passes are now running within all of her responses. She seems to associate this with the fact that she has been part of a large family, in which there have often been young children to look after. At this point, she appears to be speaking from the perspective of her own childhood, when her mother was still alive. Participant 3 then reveals a little more about her personal relationship with music when asked about her religion.

Sam: *And how about your religion? What's your religion?*

Participant 3: *Oh, that was there. [Sings something under her breath]. At night before we went to bed. My family were very keen on religion. They still are.*[102]

The memory of the religious song that was sung to her before bed as a child has remained in Participant 3's memory, although it is not clear who it was that would sing the song. There is then a creeping sense of sadness as the interview starts to draw to a close.

Sam: *And, in your opinion, what's the most important quality in a...*

Participant 3: *What's a what?*

Sam: *...the most important quality in a human being? You've said a lot that people being hard working is important. Is there anything else that you think is important?*

Participant 3: *We were very happy. We grew up. Some of us moved away, but we always came home. On our bikes. We didn't have cars when we were young.*[103]

Once again, Participant 3 does not answer my question directly, choosing instead to reiterate that she had a happy upbringing. Her mention of returning home comes again in the final words of the interview, with a slightly different context.

Sam: *And what are your hopes for the future?*

Participant 3: *My hopes for the future are very few. I'm getting old. [Long pause].*

Sam: *And this is quite a tricky question, but if you were going to look back over your life and try to imagine it as a story, what do you think the message, or the theme of the story would be?*

Participant 3: *My mum and dad were always happy. I mean, we now and then got a slap, but not very often. And that kind of thing. The animals were always very happy.*

Sam: *Well, thank you so much for talking to me today, it's been really, really lovely to speak with you.*

Participant 3: *It was a happy childhood. Now they're growing up. But it's still happy. I just came from home this morning.*[104]

Although Participant 3 has been in a positive mood throughout the interview, she has become increasingly confused as it has progressed. She has lived in the nursing home for a number of years, but she seems to be completely unaware that it is her home, believing instead that she is simply visiting for the day.

The predominant thing that I took from my first session with Participant 3 was the complicated relationship that she had with time ("But the trouble was we grew up so quickly" and "I never had enough time.") and how this relationship had an impact on her storytelling style. I was able to piece together a narrative path from her responses, but the blurring of lines between stories from different generations, all of which were defined and punctuated by children and babies, meant that it was difficult to understand the timeline of the experiences that she was sharing. I wondered whether the pressure to provide me with a linear narrative throughout our first session had led Participant 3 to become more confused, so I decided to give Participant 3 an opportunity to talk about her life in a different way, without the pressure of trying to remember which period of her life she was talking about. Therefore, for her second session, I planned a word association task in which I asked her to respond to single words.

There is a sad mood at the beginning of the second session with Participant 3.[105]

Sam: *OK, this is participant number 3, session 2. OK, what does the word life mean to you?*

Participant 3: *What?*

Sam: *What does the word life mean to you?*

Participant 3: *Oh, the last month, it's been nothing. I come in here and sit. And then wait. It gets better then it doesn't.*[106]

Just as at the end of session 1, Participant 3 seems confused about her surroundings. It is a surprise to find her in this low mood and it feels as though she is not in her usual dreamlike state at this moment and is, therefore, more aware of what is going on, which is distressing for her. However, her mood brightens at the mention of children, and she reverts to her hypnogogic storytelling style.

Sam: *What does the word children mean to you?*

Participant 3: *[Suddenly happier] Ah, that's a different question. They're my buddies. I've got six in one little flock, and five in another. They're always on the doorstep.*
Sam: *And do you like being around the children?*
Participant 3: *They're my babies. [Pause].*[107]

What is fascinating here is Participant 3's use of the word "flock" when describing a group of children. The affectionate use of farming language suggests that (a) her relationship with children may extend to her relationship with animals, and (b) that this feeling of affection for the group of children is reminiscent of feelings that she may have had during her childhood when she lived on the farm. Participant 3 then seems to become confused about time when asked about the words, 'mother' and 'father'.

Sam: *What does the word family mean to you?*
Participant 3: *Everything.*
Sam: *How about the word mother?*
Participant 3: *Ah, that's important. [Pause].*
Sam: *Why is it important?*
Participant 3: *[Pauses for a long time to think but says nothing].*
Sam: *How about the word father?*
Participant 3: *Oh, he's always there. He's a good father.*[108]

Participant 3 is deep in thought at the mention of the word, 'mother'. She is clear in her thinking that she believes the word to be important, but she cannot think of another way to articulate why this is, despite thinking about it for some time. However, when the word, 'father' is mentioned, she seems to fall backwards into a time when her father was alive. She then starts to talk about children again, although she is unsure of her relationship to them, or how many of them there are.

Sam: *These are a bit different. How about happiness? What does the word happiness mean?*
Participant 3: *[Unrecognisable speech] They tell you what to do and what not to do.*
Sam: *And what makes you feel happy?*
Participant 3: *The little ones. I've got five small ones and six bigger ones. They keep me busy.*
Sam: *Are they your children or your grandchildren?*
Participant 3: *They are more, more my children.*[109]

It is curious that when Participant 3 talks about children, she always mentions how many of them there are. However, the numbers are always different. She then goes on to mention the loss of her brother, as she did in session 1.

Sam: *And how about the word sadness? What does the word sadness mean to you?*
Participant 3: *Oh, I have my share of that. I lost my favourite brother.*[110]

She says this with complete conviction, which is in contrast to the introspective and dreamlike manner to which she has responded to the last few words. This loss, which she talks about in more detail in session 1, has clearly been extremely traumatic for Participant 3, and there is a sense that it sits within a different memory bank to the other information that she shares with me. She then begins to talk about children again.

Sam: *And how about the word love? What does the word love mean to you?*
Participant 3: *Everything. The children, and my family.*[111]

Before revealing a little about how the passing of time causes her confusion.

Sam: *And how about the word time? What does the word time mean to you?*
Participant 3: *Not a lot. I come in in the morning and at breakfast. And then whatever on the night. And we had lunch. Nothing very exciting.*[112]

These comments are similar to those that she made at the end of the first session, and at the beginning of the second session. Despite not leaving her room, and having been a resident of the nursing home for several years, Participant 3 does not believe that she is at 'home' and instead seems to think that she is a visitor that comes for the day. The fact that she is surrounded by 'familiar' objects (photographs, the stuffed cat) does not seem to have a positive impact on how she connects to the space in which she lives. I then attempt to push the boundaries of what Participant 3 might like to tell me.

Sam: *And what about the word art? What does the word art mean to you?*
Participant 3: *Not a lot. I have my little ones, and they say, "Can I come and help you?" And that's always nice.*[113]

Participant 3 is not comfortable answering this question, and so changes the subject back to children. At this point, I begin to wonder whether these conflicting 'memories' of children really are 'real' memories. The lack of information that Participant 3 can remember about her experience of raising children suggests that these recollections could be a deflective device that she uses when she is unable to answer a question due to her memory loss. I am then very surprised by what Participant 3 is able to tell me next.

Sam: *And how about the word silence? What does the word silence mean to you?*
Participant 3: *Simon?*
Sam: *Silence.*

Participant 3: *I haven't got any Simons. I've got ******* [the brother that died at a young age] and *****. Oh, there's so many of them. Fifteen of them.*

Sam: *And what about the word memory? What does the word memory mean to you?*

Participant 3: *Lots of family. We had a happy family.*[114]

Here, Participant 3 has misheard me, because there was some loud building work happening outside her bedroom window. However, what is interesting here is her ability to remember the names of two of her brothers, one of whom has not been mentioned until this point. She then mentions that there were fifteen of them, presumably referring to her siblings, although this is not clear. Finally, I asked her about the word dream.

Sam: *And what about the word dream? What does the word dream mean to you?*

Participant 3: *Not a lot. I never have time.*[115]

Participant 3 spends much of her time dreaming, so this is an interesting insight into the way in which she experiences the world. It is also of interest that she mentions time (or lack of it) again, and I wonder if this is to do with her awareness that she may be coming to the end of her life. I then attempt to end the session, but Participant 3 continues to speak.

Sam: *Well, that's wonderful. Thank you so much for talking to me this morning.*

Participant 3: *We have a little farm. And there's always something going on. I would follow chickens and turkeys and geese.*[116]

The change in tense here suggests, once again, that Participant 3 is confused about the timeline of these moments in her life. Curiously, the session ends as follows:

Sam: *Speaking of turkeys, I can see from your reindeer socks that you like Christmas. What does Christmas mean to you?*

Participant 3: *Lovely. I am fifteen years old.*

Sam: *Well, we'll stop that there. Thank you so much for talking to me. I really appreciate your time.*[117]

Here, Participant 3 tells me that she is "fifteen years old" I have not asked her age, but she seems to want to share this information with me. In this session, Participant 3 has drifted between different moments in time and has demonstrated that she is able to inhabit several identities from several periods of her life, at once. The tone of her voice has changed between the dreamier and more lucid moments, and her mood is noticeably happier when she is able to share memories from different times in her life without the pressure of the need for a narrative timeline. However, in both session 1 and session 2, Participant 3 appears to revert to 'stock answers' (mainly about children, her childhood, work ethic, and time), and I wonder whether the use of environmental sounds might trigger some more specific memories about Participant 3's past.

I begin session 3 by playing some environmental farm sounds to Participant 3.[118]

Sam:	*So, this is Participant 3, Session 3. OK, we're going to start by listening to some sounds, which you might recognise.*

[Sam and Participant 3 listen to some environmental farm sounds. The sounds include chickens, cows, sheep, and geese].

Sam:	*What do you think those sounds were?*
Participant 3:	*I've got no idea.*
Sam:	*Do they remind you of anything?*
Participant 3:	*No. They were all before my day.*[119]

I am surprised that Participant 3 does not recognise the environmental sounds. I am also surprised by her comment that, "They were all before my day" as this is the first time that Participant 3 has mentioned a past that existed before her own childhood. I then ask some more questions, to see if the sounds have triggered any memories for Participant 3.

Sam:	*All before your day... and so... do you want me to tell you what they were?*
Participant 3:	*Yes.*
Sam:	*So, those sounds were recordings from a farm.*
Participant 3:	*A what?*
Sam:	*Of a farm. So, there were sounds of sheep and chickens and I was wondering if that triggered any memories for you?*
Participant 3:	*The chickens, yes.*
Sam:	*Did you recognise the chicken?*
Participant 3:	*No.*
Sam:	*You didn't, in the recording? That's fine, that's OK.*[120]

Participant 3 is adamant that she has not recognised the sounds from the recording, even when I reveal to her what they were. Interestingly, she is also not responding in her dreamlike state, but seems more connected with the conversation, in the way that she has been each time that she has shared the story of her brother's death. Participant 3 then begins to talk about the farm.

Participant 3:	*We had a little farm.*
Sam:	*And what was it like, growing up on the farm?*
Participant 3:	*Oh, it was fun.*

Sam: *What was fun about it?*
Participant 3: *Hard work. You didn't get a choice. You had to get out there and get it done.*[121]

This is very similar to the information that Participant 3 has shared before about her childhood on the farm. However, she then starts to give a little more detail which she has not mentioned in sessions one or two.

Sam: *And what were your responsibilities on the farm?*
Participant 3: *Oh, helping.*
Sam: *And what did you like doing best? What was your favourite thing to do?*
Participant 3: *Ooh, wheeling the hay. That was always most exciting.*
Sam: *And which of the animals did you enjoy helping with the most?*
Participant 3: *The horse.*
Sam: *The horse.*
Participant 3: *[Unrecognisable speech] You got on with it.*
Sam: *And what did you used to do to help with the horse?*
Participant 3: *Wheel the turf in... we did what we had to do. You weren't told what to do, you did what was there to be done.*[122]

Participant 3 is becoming more lucid by this point in the conversation and is sharing what feels like actual details from her childhood, rather than her collection of 'stock answers' about not having enough time, working hard, and looking after children, that she has shared so far in sessions 1 and 2. She then displays a sense of humour, when she mentions cows.

Sam: *And were there any other animals that you enjoyed looking after?*
Participant 3: *The cows. I used to keep out of their way.*
Sam: *Why did you keep out of the cows' way?*
Participant 3: *Because they chased you.*
Sam: *[Laughing] Oh my goodness!*[123]

This is a turning point in the conversation. Participant 3's ability to share an amusing anecdote about being chased by cows demonstrates a level of social intelligence that she has not been able to show until this moment, and it also creates a moment of human connection between the two of us through our mutual laughter. However, this moment of connection and increased lucidity is interrupted by the nursing home environment.

Sam: *What's your favourite memory of being on the farm?*

[There is lots of background noise at this point. Care workers can be heard laughing in the background and there are roadworks happening on the street outside].

Participant 3:	*[Unrecognisable speech] You didn't have a memory. You were sent out to get on with it.*[124]

At this moment in the interview the environment becomes extremely loud and unpleasant, which seems to lead to some confusion for Participant 3. She reverts to her dreamlike state when she says, "You didn't have a memory" which she then follows with one of her stock answers of, "You were sent out to get on with it." Curiously, when the noise begins to calm down (particularly the noise *inside* the care home of laughing care workers) Participant 3 then seems to return to her period of lucidity and is able to share more specific details about her family.

Sam:	*And how old were you when you lived on the farm?*
Participant 3:	*How old? Until I went to work.*
Sam:	*So it was when you were a child?*
Participant 3:	*Yes. At seven. Mind you, you had to do it properly. He was a good dad.*
Sam:	*And who did you live on the farm with?*
Participant 3:	*Who did I live on the farm with?*
Sam:	*Mmmhmm.*
Participant 3:	*The family.* ***** *was the oldest, and* ***** *was next.* **** *was next, and* ****. **** *was a lot younger than me. It was a good life.*
Sam:	*And did all of your siblings work on the farm until you went out to work?*
Participant 3:	*Yes. We had no option. We had to earn some money.*[125]

Here, Participant 3 has remembered the age that she was when she started working on the farm, and the names of three of her brothers. This is the first time that she has demonstrated the ability to share actual facts about her family, other than the details of the death of her brother. She then shares a traumatic memory that she has not mentioned before.

Sam:	*[Pointing to a black and white photograph on the wall] Is this a picture of your brother on the wall?*
Participant 3:	*Yes.*
Sam:	*And what was his name?*
Participant 3:	*He was* ****.
Sam:	****.
Participant 3:	*He was shot. They said he had done something that he didn't.* ***** *said he had never seen the thing... [unrecognisable speech]. They shot him so that he couldn't deny it. There was no respect for a life then.*[126]

Participant 3 has talked about the loss of her "favourite brother" on several occasions during our previous sessions. However, this information about another, hidden brother that was killed is new and is told in some detail. At this point in the conversation, she is still speaking with conviction. She then continues to talk in more specific detail about her childhood.

Sam: _And whereabouts did you live at that time? Where was the farm?_
Participant 3: _Eh?_
Sam: _Where was the farm?_
Participant 3: _Where it is now. The same place. My poor old mum, she worked so hard. She had fourteen kids._
Sam: _Fourteen! My goodness!_
Participant 3: _Fourteen. But she was always cheerful._
Sam: _Did your mum like being on the farm?_
Participant 3: _We never asked her. She never had an option. There was nothing else to do._
Sam: _And what was your mum like?_
Participant 3: _Mum was good. Strong._[127]

This is a departure from the way in which Participant 3 has talked about her childhood in sessions one and two. Not only is she able to tell me how many siblings she had, but she is also able to think of a way to describe her mother, which she was not about to do when asked about her during session 2. Participant 3 seems pleased that she has been able to remember this information, but then, with this increased lucidity, comes a moment of contemplation.

Sam: _Is there a memory from your childhood that really stands out as being really important or significant?_
Participant 3: _Yes, lots of different things have passed by and I've forgotten about them._[128]

Even though Participant 3 has been able to tell me many more memories during this session, that brings with it an awareness that there are still many things that she cannot remember, which lowers her mood. She deflects this by once again demonstrating her sense of humour.

Sam: _And how about in your later... in your adult life? Did you marry?_
Participant 3: _I did. I was a right tearaway._
Sam: _[Laughing] Why were you a tearaway? What did you do?_
Participant 3: _All things, out of sight!_[129]

Here, Participant 3 is showing her ability to judge a social situation. She knows that calling herself a "tearaway" will make me laugh, and there is a sense that there are more memories that she is choosing to keep to herself at this moment. This ability to 'hold back' some of her memories shows that (a) at this moment she has many to choose from, (b) she is in control of what she chooses to share with me, and (c) she has an awareness of the impact that 'keeping me guessing' will have upon the dynamic between the two of us. Participant 3 continues to share more new information with me as the conversation comes to an end, but she is interrupted by a loud noise from outside, which seems to interrupt her train of thought.

Sam:	*And how about children? Did you have children?*
Participant 3:	*Lots of children. Dozens of them.*
Sam:	*And what about grandchildren?*
Participant 3:	*I've got three grandchildren. **** and I mostly grew up together. And then the war. [The building work outside makes a sudden, very loud bang. It sounds like a scaffolding pole dropping to the floor]. Was that you?*
Sam:	*No, that was outside.*
Participant 3:	*It was outside.*
Sam:	*Yes, there's some building work going on outside. Well, that's wonderful. Well, it's so lovely to talk to you this morning, as always. Thank you for sharing some memories about the farm. It's been lovely to talk to you.*
Participant 3:	*I didn't know anything else. It was all effort. Chasing the cows and the sheep.*
Sam:	*And you enjoyed it?*
Participant 3:	*Oh, I had no option. They didn't ask me if I enjoyed it. I was sent there to do the job and I had to do it.*
Sam:	*Well, thank you so much for talking to me. It's been lovely to talk to you.*[130]

This is the first time that Participant 3 has been able to tell me with confidence how many great-grandchildren she has, and the way that she delivers it makes it seem believable. However, the noise outside unsettles her, and she slips back into her dreamlike state, stating more of her stock phrases about her childhood on the farm, and the work ethic of her family.

What fascinated me about my third session with Participant 3 was that, although she did not recognise any of the sounds from the farm when I played her the environmental noise, it did seem to trigger a period of increased lucidity, and she was able to access more memories than she was able to during our previous sessions. However, it is not clear whether (a) this is a direct impact of the environmental noise which Participant 3 was able to identify on an unconscious level or (b) her brain has processed the sounds in the same way that the brain processes music, thus producing the same outcome of increased lucidity. In terms of the reaction to sounds, however, what is of note is that the environmental noise of the nursing home and the sounds in the street outside interrupted Participant 3's ability to access memories and encouraged her to enter back into her dreamlike state, which is evident both in the words that she says and in the sound quality of her voice.

For Participant 3's fourth session, I decided to try two things.[131] Firstly, I wanted to start the session by showing her some images of sheep, chickens, hay bales, and cows, so I could compare her reaction to visual and aural prompts. I also wanted to see if I could empower her by putting her in the position of 'teacher'. I have no experience of working on a farm, and I wanted to see if being given the opportunity to share her knowledge would lift her mood.

Participant 3 begins the session in her typical dreamlike state.

Sam: *Thank you. So, as I just said, ********, I've got some photographs here today that I wanted to show you.*
Participant 3: *Yes.*
Sam: *And I wanted to just have a look at them first. These are the first two pictures. [Sam hands Participant 3 an A4 piece of paper. In the top half of the piece of paper is a photograph or some chickens. On the bottom half of the piece of paper is a photograph of some sheep].*
Participant 3: *I better have my glasses.*
Sam: *You need your glasses? Shall I pass them to you? [Picks up some reading glasses from the overbed table] Are they these ones here? [Passes them to Participant 3] Got them?*
Participant 3: *Thank you.*
Sam: *That's OK.*

[Participant 3 looks at the two images for a long time]

Sam: *So, do you recognise either of those images?*
Participant 3: *The chickens. I'm always chasing the chickens. [Long pause as she continues to study the two images].*
Sam: *How about the bottom one?*
Participant 3: *I didn't know what that was. [Long pause as she continues to study the two images].*[132]

After taking some time to study the two images, Participant 3 is able to recognise the photograph of the chickens, which she talks about in the present tense. However, despite studying the images for a long time, she is unable to recognise the photograph of the sheep. She also struggles to identify the images on the second piece of paper.

Sam: *Would you like to have a look at the other pictures as well? I've got two pictures on this sheet too. [Sam passes Participant 3 another sheet of A4 paper. In the top half of the piece of paper is a photograph of some hay bales. On the bottom half is a photograph of some cows].*
Participant 3: *Thank you.*
Sam: *That's OK.*

[Participant 3 looks at the two images for a long time]

Sam:	*Is there anything that looks familiar on that page?*
Participant 3:	*No, I don't understand any of those.*[133]

It is surprising that, of the four images, Participant 3 is only able to identify the photograph of the chickens, but the fact that she spends so long looking at them suggests that she might recognise them on some level. However, she is adamant that she does not "understand" what the images are. I then give Participant 3 an opportunity to share some of her experiences of living on the farm, and her responses are dreamy but precise.

Sam:	*That's OK. So, on the first sheet, you recognised that the top picture was of some chickens. Did you used to look after chickens when you lived on the farm?*
Participant 3:	*All the time. They were always under my feet.*
Sam:	*[Laughing] And what can you remember... because I've never looked after chickens. What can you remember about how to look after chickens? What could you tell me about it?*
Participant 3:	*Well, feed them and give them drink.*
Sam:	*What do they eat?*
Participant 3:	*There was always chickens running around and turkeys...*
Sam:	*Turkeys, as well?*
Participant 3:	*Turkeys and geese.*[134]

Participant 3 seems to be enjoying telling me about her time on the farm and taking the role of 'expert' within our conversation seems to lift her mood. She then enjoys sharing an anecdote about selling turkeys at Christmas.

Participant 3:	*Oh, the geese were cruel. Keep out of the geese's way. We had to hold our turkeys to be vaccinated, or whatever you called it. My mum had a thing about turkeys.*
Sam:	*When you say she had a thing about turkeys, did she like them?*
Participant 3:	*She liked them.*
Sam:	*What was it she liked about them?*
Participant 3:	*Just before Christmas, we plucked them and took them to town and sold them for Christmas dinner. Some of them came to America.*
Sam:	*Wow.*
Participant 3:	*It was a busy day.*[135]

This conversation feels very different from the other three sessions that I have had with Participant 3. Not only does she seem to be enjoying sharing her memories, but she is consistently staying within the past tense when sharing her recollections, and she seems to have found a happy balance in her storytelling style in which she is able to clearly articulate herself whilst still staying within her comfortable, dreamlike state. Later in the conversation, Participant 3 shares some further memories about her life on the farm.

Sam: *And were there any other animals that you looked after on the farm?*
Participant 3: *Oh yes, calves and lambs. The lot! Anything that walked, we looked after it!*
Sam: *And what did you enjoy looking after the most? Which animal was your favourite?*
Participant 3: *Oh, the sheep. They used to run like hell across the mountain.*
Sam: *And what did you have to do to look after the sheep?*
Participant 3: *Feed them, the rotten things! Then they followed you home for more. They were always hungry. And ducks...*
Sam: *And ducks as well?*
Participant 3: *Ducks as well. Turkeys, ducks and geese.*
Sam: *Wow. And did you grow any crops?*
Participant 3: *Any?*
Sam: *Did you grow any crops? Fruit and vegetables or...*
Participant 3: *If you didn't have the vegetables, you didn't have the chicken. Or the turkeys. You had to have the vegetables.*[136]

Participant 3's anecdote about the sheep is of particular interest here, as she is not able to identify the sheep in the photograph that I showed her, but she is able to remember how the sheep used to behave and can explain it in an articulate and humorous way. She seems to have found her role of teacher empowering, and her mood has improved. As the conversation comes to an end, however, Participant 3 begins to lose some of her increased lucidity and drifts back into a state which is more typical of her usual demeanour.

Sam: *And so, did you grow the vegetables to feed to the chickens?*
Participant 3: *They were boys.*
Sam: *They were all boys?*
Participant 3: *They were cocks. That was their favourite time of day.*
Sam: *And what was your favourite job to do on the farm?*
Participant 3: *Oh, you weren't asked what was your favourite. You just got on with whatever needed to be done.*
Sam: *Well, thank you so much. As I said at the beginning, [before the recording started] I've got no experience at all of being on a farm or working on a farm, so it's been really interesting to listen to what you've had to say and to learn from you this morning.*
Participant 3: *Oh, you do. You got sent home.*
Sam: *Well, thank you very much. As always, it's really lovely to talk to you.*[137]

There is a change here. Although Participant 3 has remained in the past tense, she has reverted to her usual narrative of talking generally about the work ethic in her family. Interestingly, the tipping point for this seems to have been at her mention of the word *time*, which has troubled her throughout all four sessions. Looking at the images at the beginning of the session has allowed Participant 3 to sit happily within her chosen, dreamlike storytelling style whilst triggering some specific memories of her time on the farm. This is in contrast to her third session, in which the environmental farm sounds (which she was adamant that she did not recognise) triggered a variety of memories, some of which were traumatic, some of which she chose not to share, and all of which were delivered in a state of increased lucidity (which she seemed to be uncomfortable with) and a renewed sense of social intelligence. What struck me most, however, during my time spent with Participant 3, was her ability to bounce freely between narrative perspectives. This shape-shifting storytelling ability allowed her (and me) to travel dreamily through time (which there was never enough of) from her childhood, to her midlife, to her later life, and back again, all within her pristine and unrecognisable blue room with the sleeping baby photographs and the sleeping stuffed cat, that she was just visiting for the day.

Case study 4

The Dying Artist: "That was lovely."

This case study begins with a letter to my late grandfather.

Dear Pop-Pop,

In the spirit of how we talk to one another now, I will stop myself from starting this letter by asking how (or where) you are, and I won't ask if you are keeping well. I'll also try my best (as I've been doing for the last five years) not to mention the past or the future. Instead, I'm writing to you about something that came up in a book that I read recently. I'm assuming you haven't read it (sorry if I've got that wrong) because it was published two years too late. However, there was a part near to the end which made me think of you, and it made me want to write.

The book is called, Klara and The Sun, and is written by a writer called, Kazuo Ishiguro, who you may have heard of.[138] *The book is set in the future and is about a solar powered robot (or Artificial Friend) called Klara, who is chosen as a companion for a young girl called Josie. At the end of the novel, Klara spends her final moments (or the end of her "slow fade") in a place called 'the Yard', and she chooses, like you did, to fade away alone.*[139] *It's a book that asks what it means to be a human by exploring themes of grief, love, faith, and rewarded patience.*

The reason the book compelled me to write to you is because it made me think about your own slow fade, which, if my memory is correct, lasted about four months, between the late winter months of 2018 and your death in February 2019. We spent a lot of time with one another during that phase of insipient death. You had lived in the care home for several months by then and there was a sudden and very noticeable change in you when it started. I would bring my son to visit every Thursday afternoon, and, instead of finding you in the lounge where you had been happiest when you had first moved there (with the two singing caged birds, the life size cardboard cut-out of the Queen and the dying lady with no feet) we would find you sitting in the chair in your room, usually asleep, with the paper open on your lap. You had been a tall and broad-shouldered man, but your body diminished to half its original size almost overnight (in one daydream I picked you up and held you in my arms like a baby), and your skin started to peel like a postage stamp that had been un-stuck by steam from a kettle. During these Thursday afternoon visits, my three-year-old son (who you called Richard, which is not his name) would prod you into life by poking you affectionately but firmly on your skinny knee, which, when standing, was the same height as his head. Once he had woken you, he would stretch up to drive his toy cars around your Zimmer frame, which delighted you. Sometimes, his small, plump hand would carefully place a car into your own hand, and the two of you would spend some time making brrmmmm! sounds whilst your cars drove up and down the metal poles trying not to crash into one another. During these moments you were completely engrossed in this activity, and the world around you (the photographs, the wall mounted dementia clock, the half bottle of Bailey's, the alarms, the lists, the sweets too chewy to eat, me) seemed to vanish, and you would relax happily into this simple but captivating game with your great-grandson.

However, visiting you during your slow fade felt very different when I would visit you alone in the early evening. On these nights I would find you just as I would when I visited during the day; sitting in the chair in your room, usually asleep, with the paper open on your lap. However, by this time of day (not that the time of day existed for you) an invisible visitor would have changed your clothes as if you were a large doll, replacing your smart beige trousers and collared shirt with a pair of crisp blue pin-striped pyjamas. Whilst your room felt increasingly familiar and like a kind of home (to me, at least) when I visited with my son during the day, entering your room alone on these evenings felt strangely different each time. The texture of the care home sound world became less dense, meaning that individual sounds were easier to hear. The alarms were less frequent, teaspoons clinked in small china cups just twice (rather than four times) with each forbidden after-your-bed-time cup of tea, and the distant calls for help were so muffled that they became harder to ignore. The light would play tricks on me, and sometimes I would be greeted by a peculiar black and orange glow even though it was dark outside. On other occasions the room would be a sort of purple colour, which made your eyes (when you opened them) look opaque and as though they were looking at someone else. The conversations that we had during these moments were sparse, and you often said nothing at all, choosing instead to sit contentedly with your own thoughts.

This period of time, when you were doing more dying than living, brought with it a peacefulness, but also a sense of purpose. As your sole (soul?) focus became the task of fading away, you became quieter and smaller, but more determined. The morning that you chose to die went exactly as you planned (it's OK, I know that you planned it), and you drifted off alone after a breakfast of two poached eggs, under a sky that was pregnant with two suns, with Frank Sinatra playing on the CD player.

I think about the end of your slow fade a lot. I wonder whether I should have wrapped you in a warm blanket and taken you to the beach. I wonder whether it was wrong of me to promise that I would see you soon when I left for the last time. And I wonder whether I should have insisted on sitting with you as you left, even though you told me that you didn't want me to, just in case you changed your mind. Tell me it was what you wanted it to be? Tell me you weren't lonely? And, finally, please tell me; what was the very last thing?

Please write soon, I'll be waiting patiently.

Love you still,

S x

The Dying Artist

I only met The Dying Artist once. She was not able to participate in the study, as such, because she had been non-verbal for a number of years. However, I was asked by a care worker to play the flute to her in her room, as she was not able to come to the lounge for any of my other performances. As I had already seen the negative impact that music had had upon a number of the residents of the nursing home, I was hesitant to agree to play to her, as I was worried that she would not be able to tell me to stop playing if she was not enjoying it. However, I was reassured that she had enjoyed listening to music during her lifetime and often listened to music in her room with no signs of distress, so I cautiously agreed to play to her.

The Dying Artist's room was like an art gallery. It was painted white, and the walls were covered with framed watercolour paintings, which she had painted herself. She had enjoyed a fine career as a painter, and her paintings were exquisite. They had been carefully placed on the walls in order to give The Dying Artist the very best view of a selection of her best works from her dying position in her bed. Most of the paintings were of landscapes in the countryside or on the coast, and some of them were of brightly coloured flowers and birds. The watercolours floated like sunlit dust above the white walls, which gave the room a vibrant and warm hue of green and blue with pops of reds, oranges, and yellows. The Dying Artist's room felt completely different to the other spaces within the nursing home. There were no dolls or teddy bears, and there was just one photograph, which was of a young man at his university graduation. It was also in a slightly quieter section of the home, far away from the noisy chaos of the lounge, which made it feel less strange.

When I entered the room, The Dying Artist was asleep and deathly still. She was lying in her bed, and her head (which had been uncomfortably propped up with several large pillows) had been turned to face away from me, so that she was facing the window. Her long, thin arms had been placed carefully on top of the white cotton sheet that shrouded her tightly from her neck to her ankles, and her narrow feet sat tightly next to one another, as though her big toes had been tied together with string. There is not a word that describes how utterly motionless she was, and her stony stillness was accentuated further by the juxtaposition of air and spin that her younger hands had painted into the trees and seas and flowers and birds that surrounded her.

Being in The Dying Artist's room scared me, and, feeling slightly dizzy, I took up my performance position at the bottom of her bed. There was a strange feeling in my hands as I put together my black, metal music stand, which looked horribly out of place amongst The Dying Artist's paintings. There was something other about my fingers as they flipped, slid, screwed, and unfolded, and the feeling of disconnect made me feel unsteady on my feet. In order to distract myself, I began to speak to The Dying Artist.

Me:	*I'm just unfolding my stand, and then I'll get my flute ready.*
The Dying Artist:	*[Silence]*
Me:	*Thank you for having me today. I've put together a lovely little programme for you.*
The Dying Artist:	*[Silence]*
Me:	*Hopefully you'll enjoy listening to it.*
The Dying Artist:	*[Silence]*

There was something oddly reassuring about her lack of response, and I began to feel less worried about being in the room. Once I had finished setting up, I took a deep breath and began to play. Skittish air bubbled hardly and roundly inside my chest, which made it hard to play at first. However, the acoustics were so much kinder than everywhere else in the nursing home (partly because there were no stuffed toys to swallow the sounds) so I soon relaxed into playing for her. To begin with, she remained absolutely still. Then, during the third piece, I was alarmed when I noticed out of the corner of my eye that her feet had started to twitch. She looked like she was being startled by an electric shock, but only in her feet, as the rest of her body remained locked in position. This strange movement in her feet continued, and then, a piece or so later, her fingers began to move, and then she lifted her arms and began to move them in time to the music, as if she were conducting. The Dying Artist continued to move her arms throughout my final piece (*O Mio Babbino Caro* by Puccini) with the unnerving sensitivity and musicality of an experienced conductor. And then, with a frighteningly robotic movement, her head began to slowly and non-humanly turn to face me. I was shocked to see that her eyes were wide open, and she stared at me with a kind of dark blindness for a short but terrifying moment. When I finished playing, she looked me in the eyes and said, "That was lovely." Then she shut her eyes and immediately returned to the process of becoming dead.

The Dying Artist was coming to the very end of her slow fade, which, like Klara and my grandfather, she was choosing to live out quietly and alone. When I played to her, she received a surge of energy from the music, and the electric twitches in her feet suggested an initial feeling of being overwhelmed. She then appeared to connect with the music, and she channelled this connection into controlled and musical movements with her hands. This then seemed to trigger the ability to think and speak, which she had not done for several years. This is not something that happens often, and when I played to other people who were coming to the end of their slow fades during my time at the nursing home (one woman's daughter told me that her mother had died many times but would "come back to life by eating one spoonful of porridge") there was often no reaction at all, and even in the case of The Dying Artist, I was told that she had not reacted to music for some years. However, what I did find was that the people who did react to music during this phase of their deaths were people who had engaged in creative practices when they were living. Interestingly, however, the creative practice did not need to be music, as was the case with The Dying Artist who was not a musician. However, her experience as a painter seemed to mean that the ability to engage with creative practice still existed, and whilst she had lost the ability to paint when her hands had stopped working, she was still able to connect with music until the very end of her slow fade. For The Dying Artist, who could do nothing else but die and swallow, the ability to be moved by music was *the very last thing.*

Case study 5

Participant 6: "I miss my mum. I couldn't make love to her because she died."

Participant 6 lived in a bed, which stood in the middle of an extremely small room at the top of the nursing home. The room was feverishly hot and was crammed full of Participant 6's unreachable possessions, which he had presumably been collecting for some time. Among these treasures was a stuffed turtle that was wearing a hand-knitted red jumper, a collection of about ten boxes of chocolates, and a large white mug which was full of black biros and had 'Number 1 Son!' printed on the side in blue capital letters. There was also a very large, rectangular glass fish tank. The fish tank contained no fish and no water and held instead some plastic plants, four or five books, and a sun hat. In one corner, there was a small television (that was always on) which stood on top of a slim wooden cabinet that contained a selection of DVDs, including several *Carry On* films and a copy of *The World at War*. There were also several very small silver photo frames dotted around the room that contained some old black and white photographs.

The magnolia walls were bare, other than for several 6x4 inch photographs of Participant 6 which had been stuck to the walls with Blu Tack. The photos were peeling at the corners (so much so, that one of them had fallen off and was lying on the floor) and had been arranged haphazardly on the wall behind the head of the bed, meaning that Participant 6 was unable to see them. The photographs had all been taken on the same occasion and showed Participant 6 in his bed, surrounded by some care workers. It looked as though they had been taken on his birthday, as in the background of the photographs, there were some balloons and a few boxes of chocolates. Next to Participant 6's bed was a brown overbed table that was missing a wheel. On the table, there was a remote control for the television (which did not have any batteries), a black biro, several magazines which were advertising mobility scooters, and a pile of books that contained word searches.

Participant 6 was a very small man, and the bottom half of his body looked as though it had disappeared like a magic trick beneath the crisp, white bed sheet that lay neatly on top of him. His fingers, which were long and hard and gnarly, were jointless, and looked almost as if they had been carved out of wood to deny Participant 6 of the use of his knuckles. The muscles in Participant 6's face had loosened to the point that forming words was almost impossible, but he would desperately try to speak, without ever needing to pause for a single breath, to anyone who was passing through. His words reverberated in a strange way, like they were connecting and disconnecting at high speed, which made it sound as though he was speaking on a telephone.

Participant 6 spent every day and every night lying in his bed, surrounded by his curious collection of things, whilst performing a ritual that seemed to be a kind of spell in which he was transmigrating into something other. This ritual took the form of some tapping music, which he played by tapping a book of word searches with his fingertips. This tapping ritual seemed to have a psychological function for Participant 6, and it would accompany his loosely formed words as they rolled and dripped from his chapped lips. To begin with, it was difficult to understand what or who the tapping music was for. However, by the end of our sessions together, the function of Participant 6's tapping music became clearer.

Participant 6 completed four sessions with me. His free association style responses in his life story interview during our first session led to a second session in which I presented him with a set of words and asked him what the words meant to him.[140,141] In the third session, I wanted to see how Participant 6 responded to music, and I also wanted to try to make further psychological use of his tapping, so I played him *Clapping Music* by Steve Reich and then asked him some questions.[142] In our final session, I wanted to see if Participant 6 would communicate with me musically, so I designed a call-and-response rhythm game, which I followed with a conversation.[143]

Participant 6's first session begins like this[144]:

Note: Before the recording started, Participant number 6 said, "I never met my mother. She died in childbirth." I was later told by a care worker that his mother had died when he was two months old. The participant also produced a percussive tapping sound throughout the interview by repeatedly drumming the word search book that sat on his lap with his fingertips. He was also holding a black biro.

Sam: *So, this is Participant number 6. So, *****, what did you want to tell me?*

Participant 6: *My Dad died in February 1967. He was fifty-nine. And his brother [unrecognisable speech] he was the same. My brother, ***, died when he was sixty. I was in a private care home for thirty-nine years. That was run by ******** council. [Unrecognisable speech] but I don't agree that [unrecognisable speech] because there's nothing wrong. They wouldn't take me in the army because I wouldn't have been no good. I couldn't run. I fell on concrete and smashed my head into concrete. [Gestures to a large scar on his forehead]. By a bomb. Shot the house. My Dad came running out and thought the Germans had dropped a bomb. My head. And I reckon that's what upset me. It took me a long time to agree to [unrecognisable speech]. I want I think, you know, one of those [unrecognisable speech]. I've been told I can use one. I've got to buy one. I've got to get someone to take me out and order one. I'll pay for it. Because the lady who gets my shopping, she comes in Saturday, Sunday.*[145]

Without any prompting, Participant 6 immediately reveals the details of two important deaths in his life: that of his father and his brother. Despite his memory loss, he is able to remember the age that both men were when they died, and he can even remember the date of his father's death. Participant 6 then begins to tell me a little about what happened to him after the deaths, including where he lived. However, this talk of a 'home' seems to trigger an earlier memory of another traumatic event, in which he fell and injured his head. Whilst he remembers that his father thought that the loud sound was of the house being hit by a bomb, it is unclear whether this was the case or not. Participant 6 then changes the subject again and begins to talk about his desire to buy a mobility scooter. I then ask Participant 6 if he has an earliest memory.

Sam: *And do you have an earliest memory?*

Participant 6: *All I want is someone to take me out in a wheelchair on the bus, because you can get wheelchairs on buses. The thing I'm after, I ain't got the money, they've got these scooters. Five-wheel ones. [Unrecognisable speech]. They've been passed by the health people so they must be safe to use, but I ain't got the money to pay for it. You know, the prices are supposed to be going up aren't they? The price of gas going up. You know why, don't you? Because we spend the money on war. And that's what I'm against. Fighting other people's wars. They say I would have made a good prime minister, better than what we've got in this parliament now,* *because I wouldn't fight in war. If people declare war on this country, I wouldn't declare war on the others. I know Hitler was a terrible man, but it was up to those people to drive Hitler back into Germany. I believe in what God said. God said, [unrecognisable speech]. And Jesus. I believe in what Jesus said. Jesus died on the cross because he wanted man to work together.*[146]

Participant 6 does not directly answer my question and instead explains how he wishes to leave his bed, either to go for a ride on a bus or to ride a mobility scooter, which he would like to buy but cannot afford. He then returns to the subject of war. This sprawling style of dialogue continues into the next stage of the interview, when I ask Participant 6 about religion.

Sam: *Is your religion important to you?*
Participant 6: *No, I say. I miss my mum. I couldn't make love to her because she died. [Pause] I've not had much. That's what one care worker said, "You've not had much off of life." Have to depend on other people to get my shopping. Don't believe in that. I think if you can get out, get your own shopping.*[147]

This is the most surprising moment of the interview. For Participant 6, who had already mentioned the death of his late mother before the recording started, the question of religion seems to pull to the surface the revelation of an unconscious desire; that he wishes that he could have made love to his own mother. Then, after a moment of contemplation, Participant 6 veers into talking about the difficult life that he has had before he begins to talk about the importance of independent living. At this point, I try to ask Participant 6 further questions about his mother, but he interrupts me.

Sam: *And you mentioned...*
Participant 6: *My pocket money comes from the government. You know what the government pays you.*
Sam: *And you mentioned your mum there...*
Participant 6: *I don't even see my money, but a lot of people say I can look after it. But I don't look old, do I? I look young.*[148]

Participant 6 no longer wishes to talk about his mother. The theme of independent living continues to develop and is clearly something that Participant 6 wishes he was able to do. Another concern of his is his age, and he is keen to ask me if I think he looks old. Next, although Participant 6 has not answered any of my questions directly, I try to ask him about his family.

Sam: *And, can you tell me a little bit about your family?*
Participant 6: *I think I've got a...I don't know who my social worker is now, but I know I've got one.*

Sam: *And can you tell me a little bit about what you're doing there? [Gestures to the word search that is resting on the participant's lap.] Is that a word search?*

Participant 6: *That lady I told you about. She gets them for me. One hundred and sixty-two. And I've got one hundred and fifty-six. That's my last one. I've got one over there [gestures towards the pile on the overbed table]. Quite a hard one. Don't get on with that one.*

Sam: *It's a hard one. And do you enjoy doing word searches?*

Participant 6: *I might get another one. When she comes in [on] Saturday, I'll ask her. But I told her to wait until my birthday, because she gets a lot of stuff for my birthday.*[149]

There are two things that are curious at this point in my conversation with Participant 6. Firstly, it is important to point out that the word search books (the one that permanently sat on Participant 6's lap and the pile on the overbed table) had barely been marked by pen or pencil at all. Their main purpose seemed to be for the use of Participant 6's tapping music. Secondly, Participant 6 seems to have an unusual relationship with his birthday, which is possibly due to his (factually incorrect) belief that his mother died during his birth. I wonder at this point if this explains the photographs of his birthday on the walls, and whether his collection of items that surround him have been given as birthday presents. Next, I try to follow Participant 6's lead in the conversation and ask him about his impending birthday.

Sam: *Are you looking forward to your birthday?*

Participant 6: *Well, I'd rather buy things out of my own money, you know. [Pause] Running out of pen. [He taps his pen on his word search three times]. I've only got one left. [Points to a biro on the table]. That one.*[150]

Although this is not the case (there are many pens in his 'Number 1 Son!' mug), I get the sense that it would not be helpful at this point to undermine Participant 6 and point out that there are other pens in the room. Participant 6 goes on to talk about his opinion of women's football (he thinks that they play better than men because they invented it) and he also talks at length about how he believes that ******** council should look after the poor. Once he has spoken about this for a while, I make another attempt to ask him about his mother.

Sam: *You mentioned your mother earlier. What was your mother like?*

Participant 6: *[Long pause]. No, I'm not. [Pause] I used to go out shopping with my dad. We used to go up to London. My dad used to take me to London and that. I've got a photograph of my dad up there. [Points to a framed photograph] That's when I could walk. That's when I was about eleven, thirteen years old. You can see the difference between me now, can't you?*[151]

It is unclear what Participant 6 means by his answer of, "No, I'm not" when asked about his mother, and he is far more comfortable speaking about his father than his mother. The photograph that he is pointing to is of a man standing next to a very young boy. It is not clear whether the young boy in the photograph is Participant 6, or not. Once again, I try to follow Participant 6's lead and ask him a further question about his time spent with his father.

Sam: *So, did your dad take you up to London?*

Participant 6: *That lady...that lady up there. I shared a bedroom with her. [Unrecognisable speech] Never had any sex with her. I don't believe in sex. A lady's born as a lady and a man is born as a man. I go by what the Bible says, and they don't mention that in the Bible.*[152]

It is unclear who Participant 6 is talking about when he says, "that lady up there" as there does not seem to be a photograph of a woman in the room. Participant 6 is swerving from one thought to another, and these changing thoughts are sometimes triggered by a word that may have multiple meanings for him. This is apparent when he says, "Never had any sex with her. I don't believe in sex" in which he veers from a comment about a relationship with "that lady up there" to a comment about his views on gender assignment at birth. Participant 6 then goes on to talk a little more about his views about war, and the need to help the poor. I then make a final attempt to engage Participant 6 in a conversation about his childhood.

Sam: *And do you have a memory from your childhood...*

Participant 6: *Apart from that, we can't keep on going to war. Costs too much money and we lose too many lives. I would like to see people help one another. I'd like to sit in one of those scooters that's got five wheels on it. Then I can try and get about. I might get out of this bed and go out and go out and go out and go round the shops but that will never come off.*

Sam: *Do you have any children, *****?*

Participant 6: *[Pause] I never got a chance because [he coughs] and I'm getting fed up with this warm weather. I'd like the weather to cool down a bit. Another thing. I'd like a change of bedroom. You know, this one for a bigger bedroom. Because I used to sit in the chair. [Unrecognisable speech] They used to get me out of bed and sit me down in the chair, but this room's not big enough to have a chair, but I'd like to get a bedroom...bigger bedroom. They've got two big ones downstairs but I don't know if I'm going to get one.*[153]

Although Participant 6 does not answer my questions directly, they do seem to trigger certain thoughts and feelings for him. War is a theme that reveals itself consistently throughout the interview when Participant 6 is asked about his childhood, and his desperation to leave the environment is another. As the interview draws to a close, Participant 6 is now only talking about the present day.

Sam: *And I you were going to look back over your life and try to...*
Participant 6: *I had a care worker named *******. Her mum works in this place. She comes back in December. She's had her baby. Last one. [Unrecognisable speech] being in touch with to help me.*
Sam: *And do you have any memories from your childhood?*
Participant 6: *[Long pause] [Referring to the activities coordinator that had introduced Sam to Participant 6] You know that man who came with you? What's his name?*
Sam: ****?*
Participant 6: *I've told him to try to get in touch with somebody.*[154]

The first session with Participant 6 was fascinating. He veered from one story to another, drifting effortlessly between the different worlds and different time zones that exist within words and imaginations, all whilst gently tapping the book that sat on his lap. Although he did not answer any of my questions directly, it was possible to pick out some of the details about Participant 6's life from the answers that he had given. However, I wanted to see if I could find out more. I wanted to know more about the relationship between war and his childhood, about the impact of the death of his family members, and about the identity of "that lady up there." His free association storytelling style had a hallucinogenic quality to it which seemed to enable him to speak to me with a sense of clarity, and I wondered if I might be able to learn more about Participant 6's life if we played a word association game together.

At the beginning of his second session, Participant 6 seems to struggle with the word association game.[155]

Note: Before the session started, Sam explained to Participant 6 that they were going to play a word association game, in which she would say a word and he would respond with whatever came to mind. Participant 6 had a word search book on his lap and there were some newspaper cuttings on his bed. Throughout the interview, Participant 6 can be heard to tap his fingertips on the word search book on his lap.

Sam: *OK, this is Participant number 6, session 2. OK, my life is...*
Participant 6: *Er. Have you been before?*
Sam: *Yes.*
Participant 6: *Well, I did mention that if they want me to get up, then they've got to find me a bigger bedroom. Then I can sit in the chair. For years I used to walk about on my own. I had a walking aid. I want to get a new one. There. Do you want to see it? [Participant 6 points to a pile of magazines on the overbed table next to his bed].*

Sam: *Mmhmm. This word search?*

Participant 6: *No, the other one. [Participant 6 points to another of the word search books and begins to tap his fingers very loudly on the word search that is on his lap]. That's the one I [Unrecognisable speech].*

Sam: *Fantastic. And did you enjoy doing the word searches?*

Participant 6: *If you turn that around a bit I'll show you. [Pause] I'm keeping this book, [he lifts up the newspaper cuttings which are on his bed] because they've got some good stuff in there. What I'm after is one of those phones. They say I can't use them, but I've been told I can. [Unrecognisable speech] I might be able to get out and do my own shopping. They can't take me out.*[156]

Participant 6 has not been able to respond to the word association game and instead shares his concerns about his living arrangements and his ambitions to do his own shopping, which he talked about at length during the first session. I then attempt to bring Participant 6's attention back to the word association game.

Sam: *[Participant 6 holds up the newspaper cuttings] So, these photographs are pictures of beds, are they? Oh, I see. So, this is a walker that you've seen advertised in a newspaper? OK. And so, let's try some other words and see what comes to mind. So, how about happiness? What comes to mind when I say the word happiness?*

Participant 6: *[Long pause] No.*

Sam: *What comes to mind when I say the word happiness?*

Participant 6: *They say there's nothing wrong with me. I can't find anything.*

Sam: *And how about sadness?*

Participant 6: *The problem with my shoulder is because my bed is like this. Look. That's what hurts my back and my shoulder. [Unrecognisable speech].*[157]

Participant 6's ability to engage with the word game begins to emerge at this moment in the interview. The long pause indicates that he is trying to connect with the word 'happiness'. However, he is unable to articulate a response and is only able to say, "No." The word 'sadness' then seems to trigger Participant 6's feelings of sadness concerning his living arrangements. The mention of the word 'family' then causes Participant 6 some distress.

Sam: *And what about family? What does the word family mean to you?*

Participant 6: *Absolutely horrendous. I used to have a [Unrecognisable speech and the tapping gets louder] bed and then my feet have gone. [Unrecognisable speech] They put me in the hospital because they thought I had Parkinson's disease. The doctor said no. They* *don't know what I shake for now. [Unrecognisable speech] They say, "Your heart's alright." If my heart's alright, then I'm alright. The only thing I don't have, I ain't got the money for, is one of those scooters. You can get five-wheel ones. I ain't got enough money. [Participant 6 starts tapping very loudly again] I think I could drive it. A lot of people say I couldn't manage one but I could.*[158]

Although it is unclear whether Participant 6 is talking about his family when he says, "Absolutely horrendous," there is a noticeable shift in feeling at this point of the interview, which has been induced by my mention of the word, 'family'. The amplification of Participant 6's tapping seems to be connected to his apparent feeling of sadness. He then goes on to talk, once again, about his desire to do his own shopping, before revealing an anxiety that he has about a person that used to visit him in the nursing home.

Participant 6: *The lady what used to come in. She hardly speaks to me now. I ain't done nothing wrong in this place. You've got to do something wrong, ain't you? [Unrecognisable speech].*[159]

It is unclear who Participant 6 is talking about here, and I wonder whether the lady that he is speaking about might be the same (possibly imagined) lady that he spoke about during the first session. I also wonder whether the lady might have a connection to his mother, so I ask the following question:

Sam: *And how about the word mother? When I say the word mother, what comes to mind?*

Participant 6: *If you asked me if I'm going to vote I'll say no. They keep on spending the money on other people's wars, and I'm against that. [Pause] God never put men on earth to kill each other.*[160]

Once again, Participant 6 is revealing a connection between war and childhood (presumably triggered by his traumatic experience of falling on concrete due to a suspected bomb) which seem to manifest themselves into his contemporary political feelings. It is also interesting that the mention of Participant 6's mother provokes a mention of God. He then seems to disconnect from the word game altogether.

Sam: *And how about the word father? What does the word father mean to you?*

Participant 6: *Do you think that ******** and **** Council would help if I could get in touch with them? I'm not asking for anything, I just want a bigger bedroom. Another thing, I'm trying to get a CD player, a new one. I've got a record player but I ain't got enough records. I'd like to get, you know, CDs.*

Sam: *And do you like listening to music?*
Participant 6: *Well, it's my money, isn't it? What the government gave me. Pocket money. Just this government is no good at cutting back on anything.*[161]

Participant 6 is usually able to talk about his father, but he is unable to at this moment. I try to re-engage him by joining in with the conversation that he has instigated about music, with some success. However, when I attempt to return to the word game, Participant 6 becomes upset again.

Sam: *And how about the word strength? What does the word strength mean to you?*
Participant 6: *[Participant 6 pauses and starts tapping very loudly] The thing is, you have got a job to do. I'm not the only one. But I've been up the hospital and they say there's nothing wrong. They're short of beds, and short of staff. They've got worse cases than what I am. [Unrecognisable speech].*[162]

The pause at the beginning of Participant 6's response indicates that, once again, he is trying to engage with the word game but is unable to. Participant 6 has no trouble speaking but seems to find it difficult to articulate conscious thoughts that are not to do with his living arrangements or the desire to leave the nursing home and live a more independent lifestyle. He continues with this train of thought when asked to respond to the word, 'children', and he then responds to the word 'dream' with another mention of God.

Sam: *And how about the word dream? What does the word dream mean to you?*
Participant 6: *Could you see about it? I don't think it's... [unrecognisable speech] God give me a pair of legs and they seem to be hopeless.*
Sam: *And, we're almost finished now. What does the word love mean to you?*
Participant 6: *I can't think of anything else.*[163]

The mention of the word, 'love', seems to surprise Participant 6, and his response is calm and articulate. The word, 'memory' then triggers Participant 6's feelings about his age.

Sam: *That's OK. And what about the word memory?*
Participant 6: *How old do you think I am?*
Sam: *Oh, I'm not sure. I wouldn't like to guess.*
Participant 6: *Well, one homeless man said I was only forty-eight, another said that I was only thirty. I'm eighty-eight now. Eighty-eight years old and they say I don't look it.*[164]

Just as he did in his first session, Participant 6 talks about looking younger than his eighty-eight years. I wonder whether this is an indication that he is concerned about coming to the end of his life, and ask him to respond to the word, 'death'.

Sam: *And finally, what does the word death mean to you?*
Participant 6: *[Starts tapping manically] [Unrecognisable speech] I wasn't made for running. I've already fell on my head. March 1941. My dad came running out, he thought the Germans dropped a bomb. I don't know. It shook the house.*
Sam: *And is that your earliest memory?*
Participant 6: *[Still tapping manically] I wasn't no good at sport. Couldn't do football. [Would never have] made a football player.*[165]

For Participant 6, death and birth are intrinsically linked, and he articulates this by, once again, talking about the early trauma of falling on his head. The manic nature of his tapping shows another moment of distress for Participant 6, and, whilst he is unable to articulate his literal feelings with words, he is able to communicate his unease with the style of his tapping. At this point, I try to end the interview.

Sam: *Wonderful. Well, thank you so much...*
Participant 6: *[Unrecognisable speech] Who invented football? The men or the ladies? I was wrong. I said man. It was the ladies. Ladies invented football. That's why they play better than the men. They were playing rugby, the ladies. They can run. I wish I could run. [Unrecognisable speech] They had a keyworker in the care home. They put him in a one-bedroom flat. Said he could look after himself. [Unrecognisable speech] They had to go in a care home because they've got something like I've got. I wish I could have got in there and look after myself. [Unrecognisable speech] I've got all the equipment. They say I was born at the wrong time. [Participant 6 tells me his date of birth] Next year I'll be eighty-nine.*
Sam: *Well, thank you so much for your time.*
Participant 6: *They say I don't look it.*
Sam: *It's been so lovely to talk to you this morning. Thank you very, very much.*[166]

Participant 6's final monologue is another example of his unique storytelling style, in which, if left to speak freely, he is able to articulate his concerns about his living arrangements, which seem to be intertwined with his fear of coming to the end of his life. The word game in Participant 6's second session did not have the outcome that I expected, as I was hoping that removing the narrative form of the life story questions might allow him to speak freely about his life. However, what did emerge during the session was Participant 6's ability to use his tapping music to communicate his feelings, at times when words failed him. The more distressed he became, the louder, faster, and more frantic his tapping became. At moments when he was feeling calmer, the tapping was quiet, and at several times it stopped completely.

When I was planning Participant 6's third session, I wanted to see if I could use music to help him to make further psychological use of his own tapping music.[167] As the music he was making was entirely percussive, I decided to play something similar, so we started the session by listening to *Clapping Music* by Steve Reich. I then asked him some questions about the music itself, before asking him some more questions about his life.

Note: As always, Participant 6 had a word search book on his lap.

Sam: *OK, this is Participant number 6, session 3. OK. As we just said, *****, we're going to start by listening to a piece of music called Clapping Music.*

[Participant 6 and Sam listen to Clapping Music together. Participant 6 visibly enjoys listening to the piece and tries to tap along to 'join in'. He cannot find the pulse and becomes frustrated so stops. After a brief pause, he tries again. This time he finds the pulse and he enjoys tapping along. He becomes more animated and his tapping becomes louder. He continues to tap throughout the interview]."[168]

Participant 6 really enjoys listening to the piece of music and tries extremely hard to find the pulse so that he can tap along. When, at first, he fails to do this it is clear that he is disappointed. His decision to try again pays off though, and he feels a sense of achievement when he is able to 'join in' with the piece. The session continues as follows:

Sam: *OK. So, did you like listening to that?*
Participant 6: *[Smiles and nods].*[169]

There is feeling of a conventional conversation at this point in the interview, even though Participant 6 is only able to communicate by smiling and nodding and cannot form any words. There is a brief moment of lucidity here and I feel as though I have his full attention for the first time. He then reverts to talking about his feelings about his environment.

Sam: *You liked it? What was it you liked about it?*
Participant 6: *Well, as I told you, I didn't know where. I'm still in this bed. I've had a problem with my feet. Had blood, y'know, from a male. This one, had another one put on. [He starts to tap very loudly].*[170]

There is something strange about this moment. It feels as though Participant 6 would like to speak to me directly about the piece of music, but the words that he is able to form are about something else. There is a hallucinogenic quality to the way that he is speaking, and it is unclear what he means when he says, "Had blood, y'know, from a male." This inability to say what he actually feels seems to frustrate him which triggers some very loud tapping. His tapping then takes on a more rhythmic quality.

Sam: *And the music we just listened to.*
Participant 6: *[Unrecognisable speech] [Participant 6 taps very loudly at this point. His tapping has become more rhythmic than usual].*
Sam: *And the music we just listened to. How did it make you feel when you were listening to the music?*
Participant 6: *I know they're busy, but surely somebody could take me out?*[171]

Participant 6's tapping sounds very different now to how it has sounded during previous sessions, which has been stimulated by listening to *Clapping Music.* His words settle down at this point, and he, once again, starts to talk about wanting to leave the nursing home. Participant 6 then starts to become agitated.

Sam: *And I noticed when we were listening to the music that you were moving your fingers quite a lot. Did you feel that the music made you want to move?*
Participant 6: *[Becoming agitated] It's no good putting a chair in this room. My armchair, I wouldn't have thought. Nice armchair. People wouldn't agree with me. Someone blamed me.*[172]

Here, Participant 6 appears to be making a reference to something that he believes he has been blamed for, which he also mentioned during his second session. The sound of his tapping is getting louder, signifying his distress at this particular memory. Next, I ask Participant 6 some more questions about his experience of listening to the music.

Sam: *And do you feel that listening to the music helped you to concentrate?*
Participant 6: *It's another thing I'd like but I can't afford it. They're on the road. A scooter made for disabled... you know, people who can't walk properly. They've got five wheels. But they cost too much... it's going to cost too much money. I can't see why the government can't pay out for it. You know, on the health scheme. This health, what we've got now should be changed. The people, I think we should change to Labour. But I won't, as I said, I'm not voting for them, any of them. Because, you know, they spend all your money on war and that. We've had enough of that.*[173]

It is difficult to describe, but it feels that these are not the words that Participant 6 wants to say at this moment. He has a set of stock responses (about his environment, wanting to leave the nursing home, a desire for independent living, war), and it is as though they spill out of his mouth as muscle memory because the words that he wishes to say are too difficult to form. When I realise that he is unable to find the words to articulate his feelings about the piece of music I move to the second part of the session, in which I ask him some questions about his life.

Sam: *And now, as I explained before we started to listen to the piece of music, I'm going to ask you some questions about your life. Do you have an earliest memory?*

Participant 6: *[Tapping extremely loudly] You can't keep going up the hospital. They say there's nothing wrong with me. They don't know what I shake for. I don't know. It just comes and it goes.*[174]

It is intriguing to listen to Participant 6 talk about shaking, which I take to mean his tapping music. Having spent some time with him it is clear to me that his tapping is connected to how he feels and is a kind of stim that helps him to process unpleasant emotions, and I wonder if anyone else has observed this. I then continue to ask Participant 6 some more questions about his life, all of which he 'answers' with his stock responses. After a while, I try again to ask him about his mother.

Sam: *And how about your mother? Can you tell me anything about your mother?*

Participant 6: *[Unrecognisable speech].*

Sam: *What was your mother like?*

Participant 6: *When my dad died that was... he used to take me out. He used to take me up to London.*

Sam: *And what was your dad like?*

Participant 6: *There's not much. He used to take me out. Really, this government keeps cutting things. I don't know why. [Unrecognisable speech] It's gone too far back.*[175]

Once again, Participant 6 is unable to talk about his mother, and chooses instead to speak about his father. There has been no direct mention of his mother since the first session, despite that fact that I have asked about her on several other occasions. Participant 6's tapping then becomes even louder.

Sam: *And how about marriage? Did you marry, *****?*

Participant 6: *The thing... one day probably will come and get me out.*

Sam: *And do you have any children?*

Participant 6: *I like to... [Participant 6 begins to tap so loudly that his speech becomes unrecognisable].*[176]

By now, it is of no doubt to me that Participant 6's tapping is a musically psychological response to the way in which he feels, and is, therefore, a very visible way to measure his wellbeing when he is not able to articulate how he feels using words. In the final section of the session, Participant 6 seems to be able to use something that he has read in the paper to form a response to my final question.

Sam: *And, in your opinion, ***** (we're almost done) what do you think is the most important quality in a human being?*

Participant 6: *I think, I think, I read in the paper if you can get your shopping yourself, don't depend on other people for your care work, or your social worker, do it yourself if you can. One prime minister said. I don't know why I keep going off balance.*

Sam: *Well, it's been really interesting to talk to you today and I really enjoyed listening to that piece of music with you as well. I can see that you enjoyed it too, so that's really positive. OK, thank you very much, *****.*[177]

Participant 6 ends the third session by veering between different ideas, "...do it yourself if you can. One prime minister said. I don't know why I keep going off balance." His storytelling quality has not changed since the first session, but his responses during this third session seem somehow different. It is as though his mouth can only form his stock answers, and the words that he would really like to say are staying somewhere locked inside of him.

Despite the ability to speak at great length, words had become problematic for Participant 6 by the end of our third session (I am reminded of my grandfather who used to exclaim, "Words make me sick!" at the end of his slow fade), so I decided to try communicating with him using a rhythm game instead, to see if a lack of words would improve his ability to communicate.

The final session with Participant 6 began with an explanation of the rhythm game that I had devised.[178]

Note: Before the recording started, Sam asked Participant 6 if he would like to play a rhythm game with her, in which she would clap a rhythm and he would clap it back, and he agreed. As always, Participant 6 had a word search book on his lap.

Sam: *OK, this is Participant 6, session 4.*

Participant 6: *At first it might be a bit wobbly because, you know, when I used to go off balance, I used to finish up on the bedroom floor. About one hundred times.*

Sam: *OK, ready? [Sam claps a simple rhythm].*

Participant 6: *And I managed to hit myself on concrete. My dad thought the Germans had dropped a bomb, but it was my head. I don't think*

I've got anything wrong with me. [He taps his fingers on the word search book]. They're trying to keep me straight, but, you know, when I'm in this bed they put a pillow like this [unrecognisable speech and louder finger tapping].[179]

Participant 6 is very keen to play the rhythm game, and when he says, "At first it might be a bit wobbly because, you know, when I used to go off balance, I used to finish up on the bedroom floor. About one hundred times" he is explaining that he might find the game difficult. Then, when I clap the first rhythm, he reveals that a bomb did not fall on his house when he was a child (which he has mentioned in all three previous interviews), and the loud sound that his father heard was the sound of him falling and hitting his head on concrete. He then starts tapping loudly, as though he is trying to tap the rhythm that I have clapped back to me. I then attempt to continue with the game.

Sam: *OK, ready? [Sam claps a simple rhythm].*
Participant 6: *[Silence, but the finger tapping continues].*
Sam: *[Sam claps another simple rhythm]. Your turn.*
Participant 6: *[Silence and the tapping stops].*
Sam: *[Claps six more simple rhythms, leaving time for Participant 6 to respond after each one. Participant 6 remains absolutely silent throughout].*[180]

Participant 6 has tried and failed to tap back the rhythm that I have clapped. He stops tapping abruptly so that he can focus on listening. He is completely absorbed in the clapping, despite being unable to respond to it physically. I then confirm with Participant 6 that he wishes to continue with the game.

Sam: *OK. Would you like to have a go at clapping back?*
Participant 6: *[Nods].*
Sam: *Yes? So, if I clap something to you, do you want to have a go at copying it?*
Participant 6: *[Nods].*[181]

Participant 6 is communicating with me confidently at this moment. He is able to make eye contact, and he is also smiling. Listening to the rhythms seems to have increased his lucidity, and not speaking allows him to communicate far more effectively than when he is using his stock phrases, or when he is tapping his fingers. Unfortunately, the session ends sadly:

Sam: *Shall we try that? OK. [Sam claps four simple rhythms, leaving time for Participant 6 to respond after each one. Sam then pauses, at which point the sound of a clock can be heard in the background.*

Participant 6 then begins to quietly tap his fingers on the word search book which is on his lap. It looks as though he is trying to copy one of the rhythms but he is unable to do it. Eventually, he gives up. After a long pause, Sam claps one more rhythm. Participant 6 remains silent].

Sam: *OK, That's wonderful, *****. Thank you very much for your time.*[182]

By the end of the session, I am really hopeful that Participant 6 will be able to join in with the rhythm game, because he appears to be desperate to do so. We are managing to communicate effectively, even though Participant 6 is silent, and I can understand that he is frustrated at not being able to join in. The clock has become a menacing counter-rhythmic presence in the room ("At the third stroke, it will be time to tap precisely") and this is why I choose to end the session at this point. I cannot bear to see him unable to tap the rhythms. It is too sad.

It is difficult to know how to feel about my time with Participant 6. On one hand, it feels as though we managed to break through his seemingly never-ending verbal stream of multiple consciousnesses to find moments of connection and understanding in listening and in silence, which feels positive. On the other hand, I feel no closer to suggesting ways in which to improve his wellbeing, other than through these moments of silent communication. However, what I did learn is that active listening to a piece of music sharpened Participant 6's mind and improved his (albeit silent) lucidity, and, in turn, when I listened closely to his tapping music, I was provided with an important insight into how he was feeling. The problem was that words failed us both, in different ways, during all four of our sessions, and Participant 6's attempts to articulate himself using prosthetic words that were right but also wrong meant that when we were speaking it was simply not possible to connect our call.

An ending (for now)

How can I bring a sense of cadence to a story like this? An attempt at a summary, perhaps. Using the mouths of five strangers I have told stories of reading, music, and creativity. I have told stories of mourning, living, and dying, and I have told stories of trauma, unconscious worlds, and *the very last thing*. Collectively, the strange words that I heard in this strange world tell the story of what it means to be human, even when our focus becomes the task of dying, at the very end of our lives. As an experience it was unpredictable, beautiful, and, at times, frightening, and when I left, I took with me an overwhelming feeling of aliveness, and a gratefulness for the ability to control my own environment. Now, before I move to a discussion of my findings, I would like to introduce *Sphere* (Figure 3.3), which has been composed using the precious words of these most unusual storytellers.

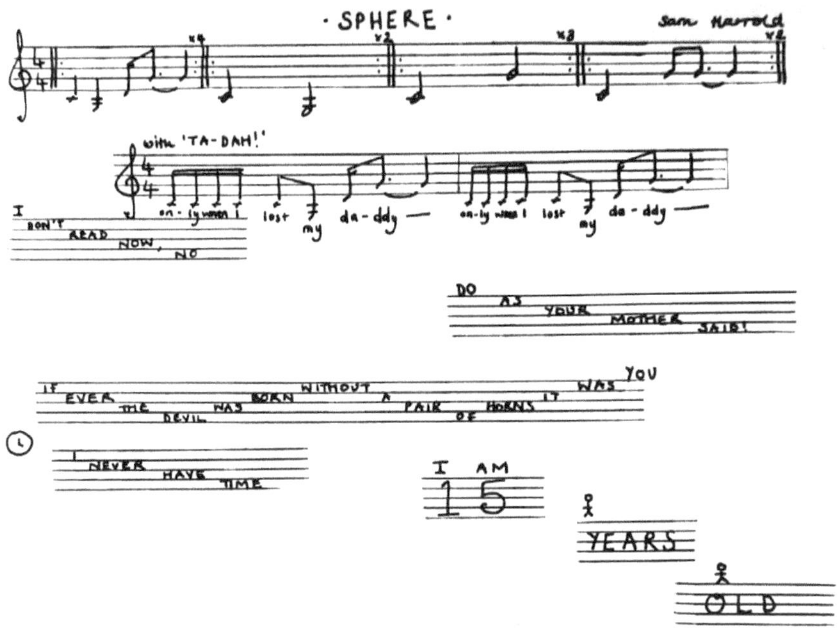

Figure 3.3 Excerpt from *Sphere*, taken from Appendix D. www.routledge.com/9781041072652

Please go to www.routledge.com/9781041072652 to listen to this and to read the score.

Notes

1 Appendix K. www.routledge.com/9781041072652
2 Appendix K. www.routledge.com/9781041072652
3 Appendix K. www.routledge.com/9781041072652
4 Poe, E. A. (1976) *The Science Fiction of Edgar Allan Poe.* London: Penguin Books Ltd. P200.
5 Atwood, M. (2023) *Old Babes in the Wood.* Great Britain: Chatto & Windus. P140.
6 Wells, H. G. (1895) *The Time Machine.* Surrey: Alma Books Ltd. P22.
7 Wells, H. G. (1895) P22.
8 Appendix L. www.routledge.com/9781041072652
9 Appendix M. www.routledge.com/9781041072652
10 Appendix N. www.routledge.com/9781041072652
11 Appendix P. www.routledge.com/9781041072652
12 Appendix L. www.routledge.com/9781041072652
13 Appendix L. www.routledge.com/9781041072652
14 Appendix L. www.routledge.com/9781041072652
15 Appendix L. www.routledge.com/9781041072652
16 Appendix L. www.routledge.com/9781041072652
17 Appendix L. www.routledge.com/9781041072652
18 Appendix L. www.routledge.com/9781041072652
19 Appendix L. www.routledge.com/9781041072652
20 Appendix M. www.routledge.com/9781041072652
21 Appendix M. www.routledge.com/9781041072652

22 Appendix M. www.routledge.com/9781041072652
23 Appendix M. www.routledge.com/9781041072652
24 Appendix M. www.routledge.com/9781041072652
25 Appendix M. www.routledge.com/9781041072652
26 Appendix I. www.routledge.com/9781041072652
27 Sacks, O. (2007) *Musicophilia: Tales of Music and the Brain.* London: Picador.
28 Sacks, O. (2007) PP336–337.
29 Appendix I. www.routledge.com/9781041072652
30 Appendix I. www.routledge.com/9781041072652
31 Appendix L. www.routledge.com/9781041072652
32 Appendix M. www.routledge.com/9781041072652
33 Appendix N. www.routledge.com/9781041072652
34 Appendix O. www.routledge.com/9781041072652
35 Appendix N. www.routledge.com/9781041072652
36 Appendix N. www.routledge.com/9781041072652
37 Appendix P. www.routledge.com/9781041072652
38 Lowell, A. (1955) *Spring Day [Bath]* [online] Available at: https://www.poetryfoundation.org/poems/42993/bath-56d221a8c0d0c [Accessed: May 9th, 2023]
39 Kafka, F. (1936) *Give it up* [Online] Available at: https://www.flashfictiononline.com/article/give-it-up/ [Accessed: May 9th, 2023]
40 Appendix P. www.routledge.com/9781041072652
41 Appendix P. www.routledge.com/9781041072652
42 Appendix P. www.routledge.com/9781041072652
43 Appendix P. www.routledge.com/9781041072652
44 Appendix P. www.routledge.com/9781041072652
45 Appendix P. www.routledge.com/9781041072652
46 Appendix P. www.routledge.com/9781041072652
47 Appendix P. www.routledge.com/9781041072652
48 Shanklin, W. (1951) *Jezebel* (song). Columbia.
49 Appendix Q. www.routledge.com/9781041072652
50 Appendix R. www.routledge.com/9781041072652
51 Appendix S. www.routledge.com/9781041072652
52 Shanklin, W. (1951)
53 Appendix T. www.routledge.com/9781041072652
54 Appendix Q. www.routledge.com/9781041072652
55 Appendix Q. www.routledge.com/9781041072652
56 Appendix Q. www.routledge.com/9781041072652
57 Appendix Q. www.routledge.com/9781041072652
58 Appendix Q. www.routledge.com/9781041072652
59 Appendix Q. www.routledge.com/9781041072652
60 Appendix Q. www.routledge.com/9781041072652
61 Appendix Q. www.routledge.com/9781041072652
62 Appendix Q. www.routledge.com/9781041072652
63 Appendix Q. www.routledge.com/9781041072652
64 Appendix Q. www.routledge.com/9781041072652
65 Appendix Q. www.routledge.com/9781041072652
66 Appendix R. www.routledge.com/9781041072652
67 Appendix R. www.routledge.com/9781041072652
68 Appendix R. www.routledge.com/9781041072652
69 Appendix R. www.routledge.com/9781041072652
70 Appendix R. www.routledge.com/9781041072652
71 Appendix R. www.routledge.com/9781041072652

72 Appendix R. www.routledge.com/9781041072652
73 Appendix R. www.routledge.com/9781041072652
74 Appendix S. www.routledge.com/9781041072652
75 Shanklin, W. (1951)
76 Appendix S. www.routledge.com/9781041072652
77 Appendix S. www.routledge.com/9781041072652
78 Appendix S. www.routledge.com/9781041072652
79 Appendix S. www.routledge.com/9781041072652
80 Appendix S. www.routledge.com/9781041072652
81 Appendix T. www.routledge.com/9781041072652
82 Appendix T. www.routledge.com/9781041072652
83 Appendix T. www.routledge.com/9781041072652
84 Appendix T. www.routledge.com/9781041072652
85 Appendix T. www.routledge.com/9781041072652
86 Appendix T. www.routledge.com/9781041072652
87 Appendix T. www.routledge.com/9781041072652
88 Appendix T. www.routledge.com/9781041072652
89 Appendix R. www.routledge.com/9781041072652
90 Appendix Q. www.routledge.com/9781041072652
91 Appendix U. www.routledge.com/9781041072652
92 Appendix V. www.routledge.com/9781041072652
93 Appendix W. www.routledge.com/9781041072652
94 Appendix X. www.routledge.com/9781041072652
95 Appendix U. www.routledge.com/9781041072652
96 Appendix U. www.routledge.com/9781041072652
97 Appendix U. www.routledge.com/9781041072652
98 Appendix U. www.routledge.com/9781041072652
99 Appendix U. www.routledge.com/9781041072652
100 Appendix U. www.routledge.com/9781041072652
101 Appendix U. www.routledge.com/9781041072652
102 Appendix U. www.routledge.com/9781041072652
103 Appendix U. www.routledge.com/9781041072652
104 Appendix U. www.routledge.com/9781041072652
105 Appendix V. www.routledge.com/9781041072652
106 Appendix V. www.routledge.com/9781041072652
107 Appendix V. www.routledge.com/9781041072652
108 Appendix V. www.routledge.com/9781041072652
109 Appendix V. www.routledge.com/9781041072652
110 Appendix V. www.routledge.com/9781041072652
111 Appendix V. www.routledge.com/9781041072652
112 Appendix V. www.routledge.com/9781041072652
113 Appendix V. www.routledge.com/9781041072652
114 Appendix V. www.routledge.com/9781041072652
115 Appendix V. www.routledge.com/9781041072652
116 Appendix V. www.routledge.com/9781041072652
117 Appendix V. www.routledge.com/9781041072652
118 Appendix W. www.routledge.com/9781041072652
119 Appendix W. www.routledge.com/9781041072652
120 Appendix W. www.routledge.com/9781041072652
121 Appendix W. www.routledge.com/9781041072652
122 Appendix W. www.routledge.com/9781041072652
123 Appendix W. www.routledge.com/9781041072652

124 Appendix W. www.routledge.com/9781041072652
125 Appendix W. www.routledge.com/9781041072652
126 Appendix W. www.routledge.com/9781041072652
127 Appendix W. www.routledge.com/9781041072652
128 Appendix W. www.routledge.com/9781041072652
129 Appendix W. www.routledge.com/9781041072652
130 Appendix W. www.routledge.com/9781041072652
131 Appendix X. www.routledge.com/9781041072652
132 Appendix X. www.routledge.com/9781041072652
133 Appendix X. www.routledge.com/9781041072652
134 Appendix X. www.routledge.com/9781041072652
135 Appendix X. www.routledge.com/9781041072652
136 Appendix X. www.routledge.com/9781041072652
137 Appendix X. www.routledge.com/9781041072652
138 Ishiguro, K. (2021) *Klara and The Sun* London: Faber & Faber Limited.
139 Ishiguro, K. (2021) P329.
140 Appendix Y. www.routledge.com/9781041072652
141 Appendix Z. www.routledge.com/9781041072652
142 Appendix AA. www.routledge.com/9781041072652
143 Appendix BB. www.routledge.com/9781041072652
144 Appendix Y. www.routledge.com/9781041072652
145 Appendix Y. www.routledge.com/9781041072652
146 Appendix Y. www.routledge.com/9781041072652
147 Appendix Y. www.routledge.com/9781041072652
148 Appendix Y. www.routledge.com/9781041072652
149 Appendix Y. www.routledge.com/9781041072652
150 Appendix Y. www.routledge.com/9781041072652
151 Appendix Y. www.routledge.com/9781041072652
152 Appendix Y. www.routledge.com/9781041072652
153 Appendix Y. www.routledge.com/9781041072652
154 Appendix Y. www.routledge.com/9781041072652
155 Appendix Z. www.routledge.com/9781041072652
156 Appendix Z. www.routledge.com/9781041072652
157 Appendix Z. www.routledge.com/9781041072652
158 Appendix Z. www.routledge.com/9781041072652
159 Appendix Z. www.routledge.com/9781041072652
160 Appendix Z. www.routledge.com/9781041072652
161 Appendix Z. www.routledge.com/9781041072652
162 Appendix Z. www.routledge.com/9781041072652
163 Appendix Z. www.routledge.com/9781041072652
164 Appendix Z. www.routledge.com/9781041072652
165 Appendix Z. www.routledge.com/9781041072652
166 Appendix Z. www.routledge.com/9781041072652
167 Appendix AA. www.routledge.com/9781041072652
168 Appendix AA. www.routledge.com/9781041072652
169 Appendix AA. www.routledge.com/9781041072652
170 Appendix AA. www.routledge.com/9781041072652
171 Appendix AA. www.routledge.com/9781041072652
172 Appendix AA. www.routledge.com/9781041072652
173 Appendix AA. www.routledge.com/9781041072652
174 Appendix AA. www.routledge.com/9781041072652
175 Appendix AA. www.routledge.com/9781041072652

176 Appendix AA. www.routledge.com/9781041072652
177 Appendix AA. www.routledge.com/9781041072652
178 Appendix BB. www.routledge.com/9781041072652
179 Appendix BB. www.routledge.com/9781041072652
180 Appendix BB. www.routledge.com/9781041072652
181 Appendix BB. www.routledge.com/9781041072652
182 Appendix BB. www.routledge.com/9781041072652

Bibliography

Atwood, M. (2023) *Old Babes in the Wood*. Great Britain: Chatto & Windus.

Ishiguro, K. (2021) *Klara and The Sun*. London: Faber & Faber Limited.

Kafka, F. (1936) *Give it up* [online] Available at: https://www.flashfictiononline.com/article/give-it-up/ [Accessed: May 9th, 2023]

Lowell, A. (1955) *Spring Day [Bath]* [Online] Available at: https://www.poetryfoundation.org/poems/42993/bath-56d221a8c0d0c [Accessed: May 9th, 2023]

Poe, E.A. (1976) *The Science Fiction of Edgar Allan Poe*. London: Penguin Books Ltd.

Sacks, O. (2007) *Musicophilia: Tales of Music and the Brain*. London: Picador.

Shanklin, W. (1951) *Jezebel* (song). Columbia.

Wells, H. G. (1895) *The Time Machine*. Surrey: Alma Books Ltd.

Wilber, J. (2018) *The Black Cat: A 100 word microfiction short story* [Online] Available at: https://letterpile.com/creative-writing/The-Black-Cat-A-100-Word-Microfiction-Short-Story [Accessed: May 9th, 2023]

Chapter 4

The uncanny, the archive, and the plastic brain

As I explained in the opening chapter of this book, my primary objective for conducting this research was to give a new and valuable insight into the memory loss experience to generate original knowledge and shape future practice across multiple disciplines. In the previous chapter, I opened up a space for the stories of each of my five case studies, and in my role as translator, decoder, and narrator, I endeavoured to provide an insight into the individual life worlds of the most foreign, precious, and secret of hidden and non-hidden personal experiences. However, whilst I have remained faithful to the ethos of this IPA study (in that the concern throughout has been with the experiences of each particular participant), and although I could write many more chapters about each of the unique experiences of the individual case studies, I must now use original readings of existing theories to discuss my findings more broadly in this penultimate chapter, to allow me to follow with a conclusion in which I can suggest practical and real-world implications for more general (and, therefore, further reaching) future practice.

This chapter will begin with a return to Sigmund Freud and Nicholas Royle to enable me to develop my earlier postulations that, for people who are living with memory loss, both the memory loss experience and the nursing home environment are uncanny. Then, I will consider how the human data that I have collected can be looked at through the work of Jacques Derrida by looking at the archival impulse, with a particular focus on how this manifests itself at the end of one's life for people who are living with memory loss. I will then turn to Catherine Malabou to question whether the creative process of archiving between two strangers (the 'other' stranger being me) can be looked upon as a form of plastic art making that is malleable, ever changing, and a kind of storytelling that takes place in a promised future space where past, present, and memory do not exist. I will then conclude the chapter by considering how the art of the plastic archive might be looked upon alongside theories of neuroplasticity, a medical theory that suggests that our nerve cells are capable of adapting to new circumstances and learning new things, including for people who are living with memory loss. This will inform suggestions for adaptations for future practice that I will introduce in the concluding chapter, whilst securing the project as one that combines innovative creative and critical practice

DOI: 10.4324/9781003639657-4

with the medical humanities and reaffirming the ethos that an identity changed by memory loss is different, not less.

A life of the vaguely familiar

> It [the uncanny] has to do with a sense of ourselves as double, split, at odds with ourselves.[1]
>
> – *Nicholas Royle, The uncanny*

This feels like the right moment to expand upon my earlier postulation that the memory loss experience is uncanny. In Freud's essay of 1919, The 'Uncanny' (or, as it is in German, Das 'Unheimlich'), he suggests that uncanny moments (déjà vu, for example) occur when something is simultaneously both familiar and strange.[2] In The 'Uncanny', Freud writes, "the uncanny proceeds from something familiar which has been repressed."[3] In other words, and according to Freud, when we experience an uncanny feeling, we are re-experiencing something that we have felt before. A repressed feeling that has been lingering in the pit of our unconscious is momentarily liberated and forced into our conscious state, before it is repulsed, pushed back, and re-repressed. Freud goes on to say, "the uncanny is that class of the frightening which leads back to what is known of old and long familiar."[4] When reading Freud's The 'Uncanny' in the context of the memory loss experience, it is useful to turn to Nicholas Royle's interpretation of the text within his book, *The Uncanny.*[5] Royle writes, "It may thus be construed as a foreign body within oneself, even the experience of oneself *as* a foreign body, the very estrangement of inner silence and solitude."[6] This sense of estrangement to oneself is exactly the thing that makes the memory loss experience uncanny and is created by the way in which the loss of one's memory can be looked upon as a kind of doubling or splitting of the self. Royle goes on to write that the uncanny, "has to do with a sense of ourselves as double, split, at odds with ourselves" and although he is writing about the uncanny and not the memory loss experience here, his words encapsulate how the memory loss experience finds itself in an uncanny space.[7] On this, Heidi Schlipphacke writes, "The uncanny feeling here is triggered by a slippage between self and other, by the blurring of boundaries between the two."[8] In other words, and in this context, rather than "loss of memory = loss of self" the loss of one's memory creates an alienating distance to the self, in which the self becomes unfamiliar, thus enabling the possibility for the feeling of the presence of a ghostly secondary self.[9] However, this is complicated because people living with memory loss experience the uncanny in a different way to others. This is because they exist in a mode of *sustained* vague familiarity.

In *Somebody I Used to Know*, Wendy Mitchell writes, "I arrive at the gates and spot someone waving to me. They seem vaguely familiar, and when we meet they tell me it's not for the first time."[10] Rather than brief and passing moments, Mitchell paints the memory loss experience as a *life* of the vaguely familiar. She writes, "If I have a conversation, or meet someone new, I probably won't remember the detail of what we discussed, just the feeling I had when I left them. When we meet again, I'll have that same feeling."[11] I experienced this many times during my fieldwork, most notably with Participant 4, who would greet me with a familiar but creeping suspicion as our relationship became more strained. It was clear that she recognised me and that she knew that she did not like speaking to me, although she was unsure why that was. There were also several times when I observed a resident feeling what seemed to be a 'false' sense of déjà vu, most notably during conversations with the three ladies in the lounge, who would often claim to have already seen that day's live episode of *This Morning*. When I asked a care worker about this, she explained that this was a very common memory loss symptom, and that these moments become more frequent as memory loss progresses.

This feeling of sustained vague familiarity manifests itself in many ways. One such example of which is a woman that I observed in the nursing home who mistook another resident to be her long-dead husband. This particular lady (a neat, slim woman, who wore tailored grey trousers and could move from one side of the lounge to the other with surprising speed) would cause a disturbance whenever the hairdresser visited, as she would insist that the unsuspecting gentleman (who spent the majority of his time asleep in an armchair) would pay for her haircut, at which he would embarrassingly search his trouser pockets for his (invisible) wallet whilst she tutted, drummed her fingertips on the arm of his chair, and rolled her eyes crossly. This would provoke much gossiping and murmurings of amusement, particularly between the three ladies in the lounge.

Interlude: hairdresser

A marital farce

The lounge of a nursing home.

Front left and facing front is a wooden chair that has been borrowed from a dining table. Old Woman sits in the chair with her hands tucked politely on her lap. She is 87 and is neat and slim with an unusually straight back. She wears a pair of tailored grey trousers, slippers, and a white blouse that is covered by a towel that has been pinned around her neck. Her hair is white and is cut into a short bob with a fringe. To the left of Old Woman stands a small table, on top of which sits a pair of scissors, a hairdryer, a hairbrush, and a can of hairspray.

Behind Old Woman stands Hairdresser; a 25-year-old woman who wears a pair of jeans and a pink sweatshirt. She has a mirror that sits in the audience.

Front right and facing front is a brown armchair. Old Man sits in the chair. Old Man is 90 and is slightly overweight, bald, and shrinking in height. He wears a pair of tailored grey trousers, slippers, a striped shirt, and a brown jumper.

It is mid-morning. The television programme 'This Morning' can be heard to be playing in the background. The doorbell rings four times during the short. The fire alarm rings twice.

At curtain up, Old Man is asleep-as-though-dead in the armchair. Hairdresser is brushing Old Woman's hair. Old Woman is coming to the end of her hair cut. She has been talking loudly and animatedly to Hairdresser.

Curtain up

Old Woman: [*To Hairdresser:*] … but that all happened when we lived on the farm! [*She laughs*].

Hairdresser: Oh, wonderful! What fun you all had! [*She busily brushes and re-arranges Old Woman's hair. She stares into the audience as if she is looking into a mirror.*] And what are the children up to now?

Old Woman: Well, they're grown up and they've moved away.

Hairdresser: [*Trying to sound interested:*] Oh, lovely! Where have they moved to?

[*Hairdresser 2 enters from stage right. She is a middle-aged woman, who is also dressed in jeans and a pink sweatshirt. Hairdresser hands her the hairbrush and exits stage right. Hairdresser 2 takes over the role of Hairdresser.*]

Old Woman: Well, erm, [*pause:*] James, the eldest, he lives in Eastbourne. He's very clever. He's done very well for himself. He [*pause:*] I can't remember what he does, but he's got a good job.

Hairdresser 2: Oh, that's wonderful! You must be very proud!

Old Woman: I'm proud of all of you!

Hairdresser 2: [*Pause:*] And how about the rest of the children? Did you say last week that the others are girls?

Old Woman: What, dear?

Hairdresser 2: [*Loudly and slowly:*] Did you say last week that the others are girls?

Old Woman: [*She pauses to think. She stares at Hairdresser 2 in the mirror. Then, quietly:*] Oh, yes. Three daughters. James was outnumbered! [*She laughs and turns to Old Man:*] That's right, isn't it? [*He does not stir. She rolls her eyes and turns her head back to face stage front.*]

Hairdresser 2: And what do your daughters do?

Old Woman: [*Pause. She stares into the mirror for a long time.*]

Hairdresser 2: [*Becoming uncomfortable waiting for Old Woman's response:*] What do they do?

Old Woman: Who, dear?

Hairdresser 2: Your daughters. [*Slowly and deliberately:*] What do they do?

[*Whilst Old Woman is thinking, Hairdresser re-enters stage right. Hairdresser 2 hands the hairbrush to Hairdresser, then exits stage right*].

Old Woman: [*Staring at Hairdresser intently at the mirror:*] Erm, your father will know.

Hairdresser: [*Not listening to Old Woman, she puts the hairbrush on the table and picks up the hairspray. She sprays Old Woman's hair with hairspray.*] Right, that's you all done!

Old Woman: [*Looking at the audience, as if she is admiring her hair in the mirror:*] Oh, lovely. I feel like a new woman!

Hairdresser: [*Removing the towel from Old Woman's neck:*] And I'll see you next week.

Old Woman: Yes, lovely. [*Turning to Old Man:*] Wake up! [*When he does not stir, she shouts:*] Wake up! [*Suddenly, and with the agility of a much younger woman, she stands, and walks across the stage like a stork towards Old Man. She taps him sharply on the thigh:*] Wake up! [*He slowly opens his eyes and looks around, confused.*] You need to pay the hairdresser!

Old Man: Oh, yes! I'm sorry! [*He fumbles in his pocket, looking for his wallet:*] I'm sorry, it's in here somewhere.

Old Woman: [*She tuts and begins to tap her foot on the floor to show that she is waiting:*] Hurry up and find it!

[*Whilst Old Man looks for his wallet, Hairdresser 2 re-enters stage right. Hairdresser 1 hands the hairspray to Hairdresser 2, then exits stage right*].

Hairdresser 2: Don't worry dear, you can pay me next week.

Old Man: I'm so sorry, I must have left it at home.

[*Old Woman angrily turns her back on Old Man, she turns to address Hairdresser 2. She is surprised by Hairdresser 2's appearance and stares at her for a long moment. Her foot continues to tap on the floor but gets faster and more frantic. Whilst this is happening, Old Man 2 enters stage left. He helps Old Man out of his armchair (which takes some time due to Old Man's age) and Old Man exits slowly, stage left, still searching his pockets for his wallet. Old Man 2 sits in the armchair.*]

Old Woman: [*To Hairdresser 2:*] I'm sorry, I think he must have left it at home. [*She turns to look at Old Man 2, and is alarmed by his appearance. She realises that her shock is noticeable, and she gathers herself. She stops tapping her foot. Quietly, to Old Man 2:*] We'll have to give her double next week.

Hairdresser 2: Seriously, it's fine. I'll see you then.

Curtain

Another very common occurrence was the mistaking of care workers for sons and daughters (please see my discussion of *The Father* in Chapter 2) and one lady would adamantly tell me that I was her niece each time I walked into the room, even though she would tell me in the next breath that her niece had sadly died of breast cancer several years ago.[12,13] Further to this, this uncanny feeling of recognising someone as someone else, which is caused by a constant feeling of vague familiarity, becomes more complicated when combined with the blurring of the boundaries between repressing and forgetting that comes with the memory loss experience. This is because the blurring of these lines creates the possibility for multiple pathways (I am reminded here of the title of Mitchell's blog, *Which Me Am I Today?* and the title of her first book, *Somebody I Used to Know*) for the uncanny to inhabit, as was most notable in my first interview with Participant 6.[14,15]

You may remember Participant 6's surprising confession of, "I miss my mum. I couldn't make love to her because she died."[16] This revelation of a long-repressed desire to make love to his own mother is like listening to an uncanny moment unravel in slow motion as he 'remembers' his repressed thought. Due to his memory loss, not only has Participant 6 lost the ability to (almost) immediately re-repress his repressed thought before he can acknowledge it on a conscious level, he is even able to verbalise it and share it with me. However, he does seem to understand the forbidden nature of his words and refuses to talk about his mother again (despite me asking multiple questions about her) choosing instead to protect his desires with a dust cover of prosthetic words about mobility scooters and independent living arrangements. For Participant 6 at this moment, the uncanny is inhabiting multiple pathways which split and multiply in stop-motion which is slow enough to provide a glimpse of the experience that he is living, and the lingering nature of these uncanny moments means that they have the potential to be even more frightening. Because of this, when someone who is living with memory loss moves to a nursing home (which usually happens following a lengthy and unsettling stay in a hospital, and, therefore, a break from being in their own home), the alienating attempts that are made to make the nursing home environment 'homely' (most commonly by filling the space with (un)familiar objects) can generate a further feeling of uncanniness, which, at best, can bring about extreme confusion, disorientation, and fear. At worst, it can render the nursing home environment unliveable.

No place like home

> Houses are really bodies. We connect ourselves with walls, roofs, and objects just as we hang on to our livers, skeletons, flesh and blood stream. I am no beauty, no mirror is necessary to assure me of this absolute fact. Nevertheless, I have a death grip on this haggard frame as if it were the limpid body of Venus herself. This is true of the back yard and the small room I occupied at that time,

> my body, the cats, the red hen all my body all part of my own sluggish blood stream. A separation from these well-known and loved, yes loved, things were "Death and Death indeed" according to the old rhyme of the Man of Double Deed. There was no remedy for the needle in my heart with its long thread of old blood.[17]
>
> – *Leonora Carrington, The Hearing Trumpet*

The months preceding my grandfather's move to a care home had been overwhelmingly traumatic for our family, particularly for my wonderful mother who was not only organising care for my grandfather but also for her brother, who had Down's syndrome and for whom my grandfather was a carer. There had been multiple late-night hospital dashes, and on one occasion I was told that my grandfather had died, only to find him sitting up in bed and smiling (albeit a little dishevelled) in an intensive care bed, having been brought back to life by a simple shot of antibiotics. When I enquired about this queer resurrection (that had taken place in the time it had taken me to navigate the stomach-turningly numberless ascension in the hospital lift), I was told by the nurse that he was given the same dose of antibiotics that I would have been given for the treatment of an ear infection as a young child. This triggered a memory of my grandfather tipping yellow, banana-flavoured medicine from a plastic white spoon into my too-small mouth (I can remember the feeling of the spoon scraping the inside of my wet cheeks) whilst I sat on my bed in the bedroom at his house, the walls of which had been lovingly decorated with pink wallpaper that was covered in a dizzyingly recurring image of Daisy Duck. The recollection, combined with the shock of his aliveness, caused my legs to fold underneath me like a marionette puppet, and I found myself on the floor at the foot of his bed.

During that particular hospital admission, which lasted several weeks, my grandfather's vascular dementia escalated, and he lost the ability to look after himself independently. When his stay came to an end and he was finally discharged, he did not see his house, or his son, ever again. Instead, he took up his new residence at a local care home in Room Number 247. From the outside, it looked nothing like a traditional care home. Instead, it looked more like a budget hotel that you might expect to see on the side of a motorway. It was a red brick, three-story building that was surrounded by neat, identical evergreen bushes, with two extremely large automatic front doors that were made of glass. Inside, it was clean with a grey carpet and magnolia walls on which there were some framed photographs of the piers in the local area. Aside from the ghosts, each room was the same as the next, housing a single bed, a brown, reclining chair, an overbed table, a television that had been mounted to the wall, and, curiously, a small writing desk with a desk lamp. Whilst there was a strangeness about the care home (I have mentioned the two caged birds in the lounge previously), it sparked the feeling of anticipatory relief that you might feel when you enter somewhere warm and new that you have been travelling to for some time and was in no way frightening.

In comparison, the nursing home in which I conducted my fieldwork was more typical of a nursing home environment, and it was exceedingly strange. Whilst each individual room was curious for one reason or another, the strangest areas of the home were the communal spaces, which housed a most peculiar selection of artefacts. Many of these relics had belonged to previous (presumably dead) residents, and these had been commingled with the belongings of the living people who still occupied the building. Aside from possessions that had been made during their time at the nursing home (Participant 9 was very proud of the woollen pom-pom that hung from her overbed table in the lounge), no residents of the nursing home were able to lay claim to a single teddy bear, doll, book, or blanket. As well as this puzzling collection of items that had been taken from residents' homes, there was a selection of decorative features that had been added by the staff of the nursing home. These included a selection of plastic plants, some empty glass vases in pastel colours which varied in shape, and various wooden signs that had been hung on the walls, one of which was painted in primary colours and read, "Mi Casa Es Su Casa!".

On the uncanny, Royle writes:

> it is a peculiar commingling of the familiar and unfamiliar. It can take the form of something familiar unexpectedly arising in a strange and unfamiliar context, or of something strange and unfamiliar arising in a familiar context. It can consist in a sense of homeliness uprooted, the revelation of something unhomely at the heart of hearth and home.[18]

This "sense of homeliness uprooted" is created in a very literal sense, by the way in which most nursing homes attempt to make new residents feel 'at home' by taking familiar things from a person's home and putting them into the new environment.[19] You may remember from earlier that in an interview with the manager of the nursing home in which I conducted my fieldwork, I asked about how they help new residents to settle in, and she said:

> We get the past history which is very helpful. Photographs, family photographs, you know, and, what else? If the family could bring in important items that are meaningful to them for their bedrooms so that their surroundings look a bit familiar. So, we have people who don't leave their room and we kind of put as much around the room that will remind them of their home. Although they know it's not their home, at least they'll see things that look familiar, a familiar blanket, that kind of thing. You know, it's just something that they might touch and think, "Oh yes, I had this in my previous place" wherever that was.[20]

This feeling of, "'Oh yes, I had this in my previous place' wherever that was" could be extremely frightening for someone who is living with memory loss, and later in the interview, she acknowledges how traumatic the move to a nursing home can be; "It's so traumatic being put into a nursing home. It's being taken out of your safe environment. Nothing is natural. This is all unnatural. This is not the norm."[21] The care manager is aware that the well-meaning practices of the nursing home are not sufficient to ease the trauma of entering a nursing home environment, but she does not recognise that the practices could be contributing to the traumatic event.

When my fieldwork had finished, I interviewed Dr Wendy Mitchell for a second time on the 12 May 2023.[22] Although Mitchell was as passionate about her work as she had been when I had met her in the previous October, her Alzheimer's had clearly advanced, and she found speaking difficult on several occasions during our conversation. When I asked her what she thought of this common approach to welcoming new residents to nursing homes, her response was as follows:

"***Sam:*** And I think the other thing about the environment that is quite confusing, is trying to make it look like the inside of their [the residents'] houses.

Wendy: Oh, yeah.

Sam: Because I think if I went into another house, say, my next-door neighbour's house, and they'd set up their lounge like my lounge, that would make me feel really disorientated.

Wendy: Yes!

Sam: And I think that is a bit of the problem. I think there's a bit of alienation that goes on there and it's well-intentioned, but actually, trying to make something different feel the same is really confusing.

Wendy: It really, really is. Because they're not at home. They may sit in a room and think, yeah, this looks familiar, but it only takes a smell or sound to confuse them because [they will think], 'That's not the right smell or sound I have in my house'."[23]

Here, Mitchell is explaining that the unpleasant feeling of, "*That's not the right smell or sound I have in my house*" (which is similar to, "'Oh yes, I had this in my previous place' *wherever that was.*") is a painful reminder that the person in question is not at home, but somewhere *other*.[24] However, for people who are living with memory loss, this uncanny feeling of estrangement is amplified because they are already occupying a kind of permanently uncanny state in which everything already feels vaguely familiar, meaning that the *further* uncanny feeling prompted by the familiar object in the unfamiliar place brings with it a prolonged feeling of disorientation and alienation to both the environment and the self. It is this kaleidoscope of multiple blurred lines that make these moments traumatic for people who are living with memory loss, and it is in these moments (which occur at the very beginning of their time there) that nursing homes become immediately unliveable spaces for people who are living with memory loss. Royle states that the uncanny is, "Inextricably bound up with thoughts of home and dispossession, the homely and unhomely, property and alienation, the uncanny becomes, in the words of Anthony Vadler, 'a metaphor for a fundamentally unlivable modern condition'" which is why Mitchell succinctly suggests that, to avoid this haunting scenario, nursing homes should be, "calm and basic. Not loads of stuff everywhere."[25,26]

Another common practice that makes the nursing home environment unliveable for people who are living with memory loss is the playing of 'nostalgic' music. During my fieldwork, I listened to an (almost constant) stream of Dame Vera Lynn, Elvis Presley, and Neil Diamond, which was played to the residents that were in the lounge with the aim of reminding them of the past. Unfortunately, this contributed to the unhomeliness of the environment. Royle writes, "At some level the feeling of the uncanny may be bound up with the most extreme nostalgia or 'homesickness', in other words a compulsion to return to an inorganic state, a desire, (perhaps unconscious) to die, a death drive."[27] Participant 4 comes to mind at this moment, and I wonder whether the music that was played in the lounge (where she spent most of her time, together with the other two ladies) triggered the compulsion she had to repeat the song lyric, "If ever a devil was born, without a pair of horns, it was you."[28] I also wonder what the significance of these words might have been, and whether the music may have contributed to her low mood, especially as she found all music (even music that was unfamiliar) difficult to listen to, due to the change to her sense of hearing, and a sensitivity to sound (or hyperacusis) both of which often come with a memory loss diagnosis. Mitchell comments:

> All these reminiscence type things… you know, there were some periods in our life that we don't want to remember… People think it's really easy to do this reminiscence. So, play this sixties music if they were born in the fifties or whatever it is, and it is not like that whatsoever. Every individual has had a life. Every individual has memories that they want to be recovered and memories that they don't.[29]

I witnessed many moments over my two months in the nursing home where music had a negative impact upon the residents, and, even if the music that was playing did not trigger direct memories for the residents (as was the intention), it is possible to suggest that the music was triggering a state of increased lucidity for the residents who were living with memory loss, opening up (often painful or unwelcome) memories of the past, but also bringing with it a reminder of the memory loss itself (which can also be thought of as a kind of home sickness, or a sickness for home), as was the case with Participant 9 (illustrated with her increasingly lucid, but desperately painful second life story interview) and multiple other people who participated in the research.[30]

A further issue with the nursing home environment (which I have mentioned previously and illustrated in *Strange World*) for people who are living with memory loss is the unpleasant environmental sound world. The alarms, doorbells, televisions, clinking of china cups, and slamming doors (which, although not 'nostalgic' sounds, as such, are all recognisable and reminiscent of a pre-nursing home life) all contribute to a highly unpleasant and exhausting sensory experience. These 'ordinary' sounds in the unhomely environment create a further sense of alienation, and in this context, it is possible to see nursing home environments as Brechtian spaces (one can easily imagine one of the white wooden signs that stand proudly on stilts outside most nursing homes to be emblazoned with, 'Act 5, In Which You Die!', rather than the name of the nursing home itself) that are riddled with moments of what Bertolt Brecht called, 'Verfremdungseffekt', which translates most closely to the word, 'distancing', but is commonly referred to as the alienation-effect or A-effect. Royle writes, "The alienation-effect is not to be pinned down and categorised, as if it were an exotic butterfly. Brecht does not specifically name it as uncanny, but the *effect* of the alienation-effect can be clearly construed in this way. The A-effect consists, Brecht argued, 'in turning the object…from something ordinary, familiar, immediately accessible, into something peculiar, striking and unexpected."[31] However, not only are these 'ordinary' sounds given a new, uncanny, life in the nursing home environment, they are also repeated constantly, at an unbearably loud volume. This, combined with the fact that the sense of hearing changes for those who are living with memory loss (as we know from Participant 4), means that the constant exposure to sounds that are 'almost ordinary' often proves too unpleasant for nursing home residents who are living with memory loss, and this is when they shut down.

When asked about this, Mitchell's comments were as follows:

"***Sam:*** I found it [the nursing home] overwhelming as an environment.

Wendy: Yes, absolutely.

Sam: It was *so* loud!

Wendy: Yes!

Sam: And it's not just one noise, is it? It's multiple noises.

Wendy: Blows your mind!

Sam: And, you know, televisions, and music, and doorbells and fire alarms and…

Wendy: Yeah.

Sam: And then lots and lots of different smells and lots of very, very bright lights. And I was just wondering, for people with dementia, what do you think the impact of that environment is?

Wendy: We shut off. I know, if I'm in that environment, I just switch off. I close down. And I'm not capable of doing anything, because there's too much sensory overload happening. We can only concentrate on one thing at once, and if we have two things happening, we can't concentrate on both and we end up not being able to concentrate on either… In a care home, I can't get over to them how overloading for the senses it is. A lot of them think, "Oh, but we want to make it a happy place!", and you're making it the least happy place in the world if they do that. So, it's so difficult. There are very, very few people with dementia (in fact, I don't know any) that can cope with the overload, that are truly happy."[32]

I saw many people that had 'shut off' from the nursing home environment during my fieldwork. However, this way of coping with the unpleasant world was often mistaken for tiredness, or an assumption that the person needed 'waking up' with loud but fleeting moments of 'entertainment'. I was told by an experienced care worker that these periods of shutting off become longer and more common as a person comes to the end of their life, until eventually, a period of 'permanent' shutting off occurs, and the business of becoming dead becomes the task at hand, as was the case with The Dying Artist. However, before this moment is reached, and during the phase in which periods of shutting down are intermittent (and not yet permanent), I observed that repetitive routines and behaviours are common, particularly for people who are living with memory loss. This was the case with Participant 4, with her repetition of, "If ever the devil was born without a pair of horns, it was you" and Participant 6's strange tapping music and repetition of prosthetic comments about mobility scooters and independent living.[33] With regard to this repetitive end-of-life behaviour, I am reminded of Freud's text of 1920, 'Beyond the Pleasure Principle', in which he first introduces us to the teleological death drive; the unconscious desire of a human organism to die, and to do so in its own fashion, or, as Freud expresses it, "The goal of all life is death."[34,35]

Freud's death drive theory focuses particularly (although, not exclusively) on the death of the self. However, it is not presented as a brutal impulse, but rather as a desire to experience the certain and total finality of the pleasurable release of tension. It is a way to return, absolutely, to an inorganic state; a state of 'before birth', or even 'before conception'. Freud discusses the way in which humans use repetition to satisfy a variety of psychological needs, using a study of his Grandson, Ernst, which he calls, 'Fort/Da'.[36] In the case of 'Fort/Da' (translated as 'Gone/There'), Freud observes his young Grandson as he 'plays' at re-enacting the traumatic event of his mother leaving by throwing away a ball of string and pulling it back to himself, over and over again. This repetition, Freud postulates, is a way of the child being able to gain some control over his mother's 'painful' actions, and, therefore, the repetitive process allows Ernst to work towards a level of mental satisfaction and acceptance of what his unconscious understands as his mother's abandonment. However, whilst this idea allows Freud to make some sense of the 'useful' use of repetition for the health of the psyche, he then goes on to consider the relationship between repetition and death. It is this compulsion to repeat (which Freud touches on at the end of 'The Uncanny' but does not unearth thoroughly until 'Beyond the Pleasure Principle') which he describes as, "the very attribute that put us on the trail of the death drives in the first place."[37,38] In other words, Freud postulates that a compulsion to repeat is an unconscious force that is stimulated by a desire for psychic end; i.e. death.

I am reminded here of Carrington's, "A separation from these well-known and loved, yes loved, things were 'Death and Death indeed' according to the old rhyme of the Man of Double Deed. There was no remedy for the needle in my heart with its long thread of old blood" and I wonder whether the uprooting of a person, (who is already living a life of the vaguely familiar) from their home to the most unhomely of environments, creates an environment that is so unliveable for people who are living with memory loss, that entry to the nursing home environment becomes a death in itself.[39] In *One Last Thing: How to Live with the End in Mind,* which Mitchell describes as her 'third and final book', she transcribes a conversation with her friend, George, who is also living with memory loss.[40,41] During the conversation, he says:

> *"GEORGE:* It's almost a metaphorical pain. Dementia reduces your ability to process, to understand what your senses are telling you, so sensory overload becomes very uncomfortable very quickly, and, for me, it's that overload of pain and fatigue that overwhelms me sometimes, and if that comes along at the same time as I'm having a tired, foggy day, what do you do about that? There's nothing you can do, but the trouble is thinking about suicide. It's one of those days when you might think: *Shit, I've had enough of this.* We're used to having days like that, but not too many of them at once, and if you do have a few together, that's when you really start to get down and look into your soul and almost say: 'What the hell is the point?' And what happens when we, with our failing brains, are unable to actually think about tomorrow being okay?"[42]

What George is articulating here is that, for people who are living with memory loss, sensory overload can become so unpleasant, that it can prompt an acceptance, or even a welcoming of death, in the form of suicidal thoughts and impulses. Luckily, George still has some control over his environment as he does not live in a nursing home, and this control enables him to manage this impulse by reasoning that the environment in which he finds himself may change, and, therefore, become liveable again in the future space. However, for people who are living with memory loss that live in a nursing home, the fact that they are unable to escape the relentlessly unpleasant nursing home environment appears to trigger the process of shutting down that comes at the end of life.

What then seems to follow is a kind of secondary death, of one (or more) of the multiple identities that come with a memory loss state, in which the process of shutting down is interspersed with strange repetitive behaviours that continue until the task of dying becomes the main activity, which is almost impossible to disturb, except in cases such as The Dying Artist, who was able to be moved by creative practices (and nothing else) during that very last phase of her life. This strange multiple death, which is made possible when a life of the vaguely familiar crosses paths with the strangest of unhomely worlds, is surely a, "death and death indeed."[43]

Archive fever

> These gloves are very precious because they remind me of last winter. I'm going to put them in my memory box, so that I can keep my memories safe, otherwise I might forget what winter is like.
>
> – *My son, Edward. Aged 8*

This book is an archive. From the personal recollections of my grandfather's time with memory loss, to the pieces of music, to the words of strange strangers, to my creative descriptions of the nursing home environment; it is all archival.

The Oxford English Dictionary has the definition of archive as:

1 "A place in which public records or other important historic documents are kept.
2 A historical record or document so preserved."[44]

And Merriam-Webster offers a similar definition:

1 "A place in which public records or historical materials (such as documents) are preserved. Also: The material preserved – often used in plural.
2 A repository or collection especially of information."[45]

Both definitions suggest that an archive must be thought of as a collection of information (called an archive) which is, importantly, housed inside a space which is also called an archive. One, it would appear, cannot exist without the other. The same can be said of this book; the fragments or pieces of information that are gathered together here (the archive) exist, only because they are housed within the book (also the archive) itself. What is useful to this study in terms of thinking about the archive is the way in which the results that I have collected offer a way of looking at the archival process in the context of the memory loss experience, which sheds further light on the experience itself.

In *Archive Fever: A Freudian Impression,* Jacques Derrida begins with the suggestion that the archival process must be rethought in terms of advancements in technological storage media, specifically email.[46] However, for the most part, the essay (which began life as a lecture) takes the form of an etymological exploration of the archive, in which Derrida uses Freud's ideas (particularly those concerning the death drive) to examine the connection between the archival impulse (the desire to preserve *and* annihilate the archive) and the human memory. Derrida writes:

> The concept of the archive shelters in itself, of course, this memory of the name *arkhē* [meaning the *commencement and the commandment*]. But it also shelters itself from this memory which it shelters: which comes down to saying also that it forgets it. There is nothing accidental or surprising about

> this. Contrary to the impression one often has, such a concept is not easy to archive. One has trouble, and for essential reasons, establishing it and interpreting it in the document it delivers to us, here in the word which names it, that is the "archive."[47,48]

Here, Derrida is commenting on the elusive nature of the archive, which he does by personifying the archive(s) into a being that is capable of forgetting. This suggests that, for Derrida, the archive is capable of the splitting and doubling of the self that also happens to be characteristic of the memory loss experience. It also implies that, for Derrida, the archive is alienating, at odds with itself, and uncanny. Later, he goes on to say that:

> "Archive" is only a *notion*, an impression associated with a word and for which, together with Freud, we do not have a concept. We only have an impression, an insistent impression through the unstable feeling of a shifting figure, of a schema, or of an in-finite or indefinite process.[49]

This idea of an archive as a process is in conflict with the common idea that an archive houses archived material which is representative of the past. Instead, Derrida is suggesting that the archive (*whatever* that might be) is housed inside the archive (*wherever* that might be) which creates an illusion of something that is 'fixed' in the past, when actually, the indefinite process of the archive (which happens because of the way in which the 'whatever' archive and the 'wherever' archive interact inside and outside of one another, in a way that cannot be separated) reveals something of a promise of a future space. Derrida writes:

> In an enigmatic sense, which will clarify itself *perhaps* (perhaps, because nothing should be sure here, for essential reasons), the question of the archive is not, we repeat, a question of the past. It is not the question of a concept dealing with the past that might *already* be at our disposal or not at our disposal, *an archivable concept of the archive*. It is a question of the future, the question of the future itself, the question of a response, of a promise and of a responsibility for tomorrow. The archive: if we want to know what that will have meant, we will only know in times to come. Perhaps.[50]

There are several ways that this, "responsibility for tomorrow," as Derrida puts it, can be considered in the context of the data that I collected during my fieldwork, particularly when thinking about the significance of the use of recording technology (a dictaphone) during the archiving process, and my personal influence over the data that was collected, both of which I shall discuss later.[51] However, I would first like to return to the nursing home environment, to consider the impact it had (and continues to have) on this particular archival process.

When discussing (what I have called) the 'where' of the archive, Derrida writes:

> It is thus, in this *domiciliation*, in this house arrest, that archives take place. The dwelling, this place where they dwell permanently, marks this institutional passage from the private to the public, which does not always mean from the secret to the nonsecret.[52]

At this moment, I would like to suggest that the house of the archival material that I have collected is located inside the nursing home, thus making the nursing home the first 'where' of this archive, and whilst the archive continues to exist inside the archive of this book, the nursing home archive has, perhaps, a greater influence upon the indefinite shifting of the meaning of the archival material. This influence was caused by the uncanniness of the unfamiliar environment, specifically the placing of familiar objects in unfamiliar places, the use of 'nostalgic' music, and the relentless and familiar environmental sounds, all of which (as I postulated earlier) created an unliveable environment which triggered repetitive behaviour and a revealing of concealed thoughts and feelings among the residents who were living with memory loss. This meant that the unliveable nature of the environment for the participants who were living with memory loss became a *liveable* environment for the archive itself. This is because, not only did the nursing home environment induce a revelation of concealed thoughts and feelings which became the archival material, but the environment also seemed to increase the archival desire in the participants.

When I was preparing to carry out my fieldwork, one of my primary concerns was that I would not be able to recruit enough participants. I had hoped to recruit 'up to ten' participants who were living with memory loss. However, I was surprised by the number of residents who were keen to take part, and it would have been easy to recruit at least another ten people. What surprised me further, was how completely desperate people were to share their life stories, all of which varied enormously, and were told with tenderness, vulnerability, and (it seemed to me) absolute honesty, even when the content was distressing or highly sensitive. I am reminded here of Coetzee's, "I want to be human, and to be human is to be a speaking animal. That is why I am telling you these things: so that I can be human again" which encapsulates the feverishness with which the stories were told, as the participants seemed to attempt to remain human.[53] This desire, coupled with the increased lucidity in the participants that was created by the sound world of the nursing home environment, and the unwelcome realisation that they were living with memory loss which was triggered by the uncanny this-is-not-my-home environment, seemed to drive this impulse, in which the sharing of life stories became a task that was absolutely necessary.

When thinking further about how this impulse manifests itself in those living with memory loss, I shall return to Derrida, who writes:

> because the conditions of archivization implicate all the tensions, contradictions, or aporias we are trying to formalize here, notably those which make it

> into a movement of the promise and of the future no less than of recording the past, the concept of the archive must inevitably carry in itself, as does every concept, an unknowable weight.[54]

Thinking again of this process as "a promise of the future" helps to shed some light on the reason for the agitation that the participants seemed to feel when it came to sharing the stories of their lives, particularly when taking into account the fact that, as well as living with memory loss, they were coming to their end of their lives.[55] In all of the life story interviews with all participants, there was a feeling that their awareness of their memory loss (triggered, as I postulated earlier, by the uncanny environment) meant that they wanted to 'pass something on' before they could no longer do so, perhaps so they might hope to 'keep living' in the future space in the form of the archive. On this, which Derrida refers to as, *archive fever*, he writes, "It involves the history of the concept, it inflects archive desire or fever, their opening on the future, their dependency with respect to what will come, in short, all that ties knowledge and memory to the promise."[56] I felt this sense of "archive desire or fever" from all of the participants that I worked with who were living with memory loss, and in some cases, it verged on an almost blind panic.[57] Interestingly, one of the impacts that this had on the archival material itself seemed to be a wide and peculiar range of storytelling styles. These ranged from hypnogogic (Participant 3) to sung (Participant 9) to free association, clothed in the prosthetic (Participant 6). There were also many other great storytellers in the nursing home, two of whom were participants in this study but unfortunately died very soon after their first session.[58] In both cases, their session with me was one of their last conversations, and both interviews unveiled a lifetime of fascinating events that were told with absolute and urgent clarity, giving a unique and precious glimpse into how the memory loss experience unfolds right at the end of life. I am also reminded here of my grandfather, who became the most magnificent storyteller at the very end of his life. His stories emerged as strange and experimental folk tales and each of them came back again and again (and again and again) in different stories and different forms, but always with him as the hero. The wide range of storytelling styles that emerge during this late phase of archivisation teaches much about the archival desire in those that are living with memory loss, but there is even more to be learned from the nature of the information that the participants chose to/were able to share. During each session with the participants of this study, I often felt as though what was being shared was a secret; a thought or feeling that had remained unseen, sometimes for many years, which brings me back to the uncanny.

As I mentioned earlier, in The 'Uncanny', Freud writes, "the uncanny proceeds from something familiar which has been repressed."[59] With this in mind, the question arises of whether the archival material that I have gathered reveals more about the uncanniness of the memory loss experience, and whether the process of archivisation makes a space in which people living with memory loss can find a place for their liberated repressed feelings, or whether what is being shared during this urgent archival process are, instead, feelings that have been *suppressed*. On repression (Verdrängung) and suppression (Unterdrückung) in the archive, Derrida writes that they:

> directly concern the structures of archivization. Because they touch on the topic differences and thus on the location of the subtraces of traces, on the subjectile of consignation (*Niederschrift*), from one system to the other. Unlike repression, (*Verdrängung*), which remains unconscious in its operation and its result, suppression (*Unterdrückung*) effects what Freud calls a "second censorship" – between the conscious and the preconscious – or rather affects the affect, which is to say, that which *can never* be repressed in the unconscious but only suppressed and displaced in another affect.[60]

When reading this alongside the material that I have collected, there does seem to be evidence of both repressed *and* suppressed feelings, which work alongside one another (just as Derrida suggests) in order to 'create' the archive. There are many moments that suggest that the information shared had previously been repressed, and although it is not possible to confirm that as fact, it *is* possible to see the difference between what seem to be suppressed feelings (or feelings that have been held within a "second censorship – between the conscious and preconscious") and revelations that, surely, must have previously been repressed.[61] To provide an example, I would suggest that Participant 9's, "Only when I lost my daddy!" and Participant 4's, "Do as your mother said" are examples of revealed suppressed thoughts, whereas The Dying Artist's, "That was lovely," and Participant 6's, "I miss my mum, I couldn't make love to her because she died" do seem to be of the nature of that which has been repressed.[62,63,64,65] I would also argue that, despite the fact I cannot compare the archive that I have collected with an archive of participants who are not living with memory loss, given the nature of these particular repressed thoughts, they were able to be liberated because the participant was living with memory loss and was living in the uncanny environment of the nursing home.

There are moments, too, where it is less clear whether the thought or feeling that is being revealed is suppressed or repressed, as was the case with Participant 3's revelation of the loss of her 'other', non-favourite brother, which she did not share until I played her some environmental sounds during her third session:

"**Participant 3:** *He was shot. They said he had done something that he didn't. ***** said he had never seen the thing... [unrecognisable speech]. They shot him so that he couldn't deny it. There was no respect for a life then.*"[66]

However, whether these thoughts are repressed, suppressed, or (what seems to be most likely, and is line with the thinking of Derrida) a combination of both, the memory loss archiver demonstrates the way in which the archival process inhabits multiple pathways for people living with memory loss, in much the same way that the uncanny functions within the memory loss psyche. For people living with memory loss, the archiving experience offers catharsis and hope in the form of a promised future which, perhaps, might be thought of as a wish fulfilled, and as I now turn to the use of repetition in the memory loss archiver, I will once again return to the death drive.

I have already mentioned that I observed many repetitive behaviours during my fieldwork. Among others, I observed a lady who had worked in a launderette who was given a pile of sheets that she would fold all day (and would become quite irritated if she was interrupted from her 'work'), and a lady who had been a seamstress who constantly moved her hands as though she was using a sewing machine. I have also already mentioned Participant 6's strange tapping music, and Participant 9, who would spend much of her time knitting endless small squares suitable for a patchwork blanket. However, it is specifically the repetition of words or ideas that reveal (or hide) themselves within the archival process that is of concern here.

Participant 4 was particularly interesting when it came to the repetition of certain phrases. The repetition of the song lyric, "If ever the devil was born without a pair of horns, it was you" was muttered in the manner of an obsession that she said time and time again.[67] The other two ladies in the lounge never commented on it, and I did wonder whether Participant 4 would have been quite as patient had it been one of the other ladies who was repeating herself so regularly. You will also remember her reaction to one of my performances in the lounge:

> When I had finished playing the fourth piece, I heard that Participant 4 was in fact saying, "It's not supposed to sound like that!" over and over again. She looked visibly distressed and refused to lift her head throughout the rest of the performance. When I had finished and was packing away, she was still repeatedly saying, "It's not supposed to sound like that" and after that Friday morning, our relationship sadly became progressively problematic.[68]

After that performance, the phrase, "It's not supposed to sound like that!" was added to her repetition repertoire and was articulated like a chant.[69] Whilst her 'devil' phrase remained dominant, this secondary phrase, which came from a place of distress at the unfamiliar sounds due to her change in hearing, was said as often as a ratio of three to one. At first, I assumed that this was triggered by my arrival, and that she was making a connection between the sight of me and the upset that had been caused by my flute playing, but I was told by a care worker that she had been saying it constantly (whether I was there or not) since the performance. The repetition of this secondary phrase seemed to provide some psychical use for Participant 4 (I am reminded here of Freud's grandson and his game of 'Fort/Da') and this seemed to fuel her dislike for talking to me about music, and although she did not repeat the phrase itself during the sessions that followed, the repetition did seem to have an impact, and she would disengage with the conversation as soon as I mentioned music:[70]

"Sam:	*So, do you not enjoy listening to music now?*
Participant 4:	*No.*
Sam:	*Why is that?*
Participant 4:	*What, looking at, listening to that noise? [Angrily, and as though she is quoting someone else] What are you looking at that noise for?"*[71]

What is also of note here, is that, following the performance in the lounge, not only did Participant 4 begin to repeat her secondary phrase (I never heard a third), she was also able to share far less information in her sessions with me than she was able to share in her earlier sessions. At the time, I suspected this was due to her stubbornness (I have previously mentioned her proud post-war mother demeanour), but on reflection, I wonder whether the repetition might have had an impact on the amount of information that she was able to remember, and therefore commit to the archive. On repetition and the archive, Derrida writes:

> How can we think about this fatal repetition, about repetition in general in its relationship to memory and the archive? It is easy to perceive, if not to interpret, the necessity of such a relationship, at least if one associates the archive, as naturally as one is always tempted to do, with repetition, and repetition with the past. But it is the future that is at issue here, and the archive as an irreducible experience of the future.[72]

In this context, it is possible to look upon Participant 4's compulsion to repeat as a kind of fatality. She, like the other participants, had been desperate to be a part of the archive that I was building in the nursing home, but it is possible to suggest that the reason that she became less and less able to record her thoughts and feelings, and therefore, contribute to a future space in which, in some way, she could, 'keep living', may have been a result of the constant repetition of these two phrases. I am reminded here of Freud's comments on a compulsion to repeat, which he described as being, "the very attribute that put us on the trail of the death drives in the first place," and I will now consider the relationship between the death drive and the archive.[73]

On the death drive and the archive, Derrida writes, "the death drive is above all *anarchivic*, one could say, or *archiviolithic*. It will always have been archive-destroying, by silent vocation."[74] In other words, Derrida suggests that the death drive functions in a similar way to the archive, in that both the archive and the death drive occur when remembering happens via a process of destruction. This is fundamental to both impulses, and I have already made reference to many observed moments in which this was evident during the fieldwork for this book. However, what is of a deeper interest in terms of this particular study, is the relationship between the archive, the death drive and memory *loss*. Derrida continues with:

> the archiviolithic force leaves nothing of its own behind. As the death drive is also, according to the most striking words of Freud himself, an aggression and a destruction (*Destruktion*) drive, it not only incites forgetfulness, amnesia, the annihilation of memory, as *mnēmē* or *anamnēsis*, but also commands the radical effacement, in truth the eradication, of that which can never be reduced to *mnēmē* or to *anamnesis*, that is, the archive, consignation, the documentary or monumental apparatus as *hypomnēma*, mnemotechnical supplement or representative, auxiliary or memorandum. Because the archive, if this word or this figure can be stabilized so as to take on a signification, will never be either memory or anamnesis as spontaneous, alive and internal experience. On the contrary: the archive takes place at the place of originary and structural breakdown of the said memory.[75]

Here, Derrida suggests that the destructive repetition compulsion which is characteristic of the death drive *generates* a loss of memory, which destroys the archive and, therefore, the self, in its pursuit of death. Derrida continues, "its silent vocation is to burn the archive and to incite amnesia, thus refuting the economic principle of the archive, aiming to ruin the archive as accumulation and capitalization of memory on some substrate and in an exterior place."[76] Derrida's thinking on this appears to align with Anne Davis Basting's, "self = memory" and "loss of memory = loss of self" which is a concept that the participants in this study have repeatedly pulled into question, and I wonder if a closer look at the use of Participant 6's use of prosthetic words might shed some light on how this idea might be challenged.[77]

At the beginning of Participant 6's second session (in which I attempted to find out more about his lived experience by playing a word association game) he made clear attempts to respond to me directly, but instead, resorted to the use of prosthetic words and his tapping music in order to communicate his thoughts:[78]

"Sam:	*And so, let's try some other words and see what comes to mind. So, how about happiness? What comes to mind when I say the word happiness?*
Participant 6:	*[Long pause] No.*
Sam:	*What comes to mind when I say the word happiness?*
Participant 6:	*They say there's nothing wrong with me. I can't find anything.*
Sam:	*And how about sadness?*
Participant 6:	*The problem with my shoulder is because my bed is like this. Look. That's what hurts my back and my shoulder. [Unrecognisable speech].*

Participant 6's ability to engage with the word game begins to emerge at this moment in the interview. The long pause indicates that he is trying to connect with the word 'happiness'. However, he is unable to articulate a response and is only able to say, "No." The word 'sadness' then seems to trigger Participant 6's feelings of sadness concerning his living arrangements. The mention of the word 'family' then causes Participant 6 some distress.

Sam:	*And what about family? What does the word family mean to you?*
Participant 6:	*Absolutely horrendous. I used to have a [Unrecognisable speech and the tapping gets louder] bed and then my feet have gone. [Unrecognisable speech] They put me in the hospital because they thought I had Parkinson's disease. The doctor said no. They don't know what I shake for now. [Unrecognisable speech] They say, "Your heart's alright." If my heart's alright, then I'm alright. The only thing I don't have, I ain't got the money for, is one of those scooters. You can get five-wheel ones. I ain't got enough money. [Participant 6 starts tapping very loudly again] I think I could drive it. A lot of people say I couldn't manage one but I could.*

Although it is unclear whether Participant 6 is talking about his family when he says, "Absolutely horrendous," there is a noticeable shift in feeling at this point of the interview, which has been induced by my mention of the word, 'family'. The amplification of Participant 6's tapping seems to be connected to his apparent feeling of sadness."[79]

In this example, Participant 6 is demonstrating his lack of ability to 'archive' his thoughts and memories, despite the fact that he is verbal and is able to articulate many other concerns that he has, that appear to be triggered by the source word, i.e. the word that I have presented him with. On prosthesis and the archive, Derrida begins with Freud's ideas concerning truth, in which he recognises that, for Freud, "there is a *truth of delusion*, a truth of insanity or of hauntedness. … But it resists and *returns*, as such, as the spectral truth of delusion or of hauntedness. It *returns*, it belongs, it comes down to spectral truth."[80] These 'stock answers' which reappeared time and time again with Participant 6 (and with many of the other participants), seemed to be far more than the simple repetition of a recent thought or memory, brought about due to a lack of short-term memory, due to the fact that they were living with memory loss. On the contrary, these answers seem to exist within a spectrum of truth in which other, more challenging memories also exist. It is almost as if the prosthetic answers are truths in themselves which serve as a kind of truth sponge which, when pushed and squeezed on top of the absolute truth, soak it up, so that the absolute truth can be alive within it. This becomes evident later in the second session with Participant 6:

"Sam:	*And how about the word mother? When I say the word mother, what comes to mind?*
Participant 6:	*If you asked me if I'm going to vote I'll say no. They keep on spending the money on other people's wars, and I'm against that. [Pause] God never put men on earth to kill each other.*

Once again, Participant 6 is revealing a connection between war and childhood (presumably triggered by his traumatic experience of falling on concrete due to a suspected bomb) which seem to manifest themselves into his contemporary political feelings. It is also interesting that the mention of Participant 6's mother provokes a mention of God. He then seems to disconnect from the word game altogether."[81]

Here, Participant 6 is making use of his prosthetic answers, which he offers in place of the literal response to the words in the sound game. Derrida writes:

> one must take into account a prosthesis, this "distorted substitute." But a part of truth remains, a piece or a grain of truth breathes at the heart of the delusion, of the illusion, or the hallucination, of the hauntedness.[82]

This 'grain of truth' can be found in the connection that Participant 6 makes between his mother and God, which he also made in his first session with me:[83]

"***Sam:***	*Is your religion important to you?*
Participant 6:	*No, I say. I miss my mum. I couldn't make love to her because she died. [Pause] I've not had much. That's what one care worker said, "You've not had much off of life." Have to depend on other people to get my shopping. Don't believe in that. I think if you can get out, get your own shopping.*

This is the most surprising moment of the interview. For Participant 6, who had already mentioned the death of his late mother before the recording started, the question of religion seems to pull to the surface the revelation of an unconscious desire; that he wishes that he could have made love to his own mother."[84]

The difference between the two responses, is that in the first session, Participant 6 was able to freely articulate a response to my question, perhaps due to the urgency of the archival impulse that he felt during our first meeting. In the second session, he appears to make the same connection between his mother and God, and although these 'connected truths' (accompanied by his tapping music, which becomes louder) are articulated differently, the meaning seems to be much the same. The archival impulse means that Participant 6 is working extremely hard to articulate his feelings, and, therefore, to contribute to the archival process. However, what seems to be happening is that something is at play which is preventing him from doing so, which was illustrated by the advancing trouble that Participant 6 had when it came to communicating his feelings as our sessions progressed. However, whilst this journey towards silence may have been caused by his increased repetition and urgency of both his 'stock answers' and his tapping music, his use of a prosthetic secondary truth that housed an absolute truth seemed to work in conflict with this apparent drive towards death, and I wonder whether, whilst the death drive is evidently at play within the archival process, its attempts to, "burn the archive and to incite amnesia" are thwarted by the memory loss archiver, due to their apparent ability to uncannily release the most repressed of repressed truths, and then hide them within a secondary truth, thus retaining an identity and a sense of self.[85] I would postulate that this can happen, not only *despite of*, but *because of* a memory loss state, during whichever phase of whichever death(s) they are currently inhabiting, as was the case with the very origin of memory for Participant 6, but also for The Dying Artist, from whom her identity as an artist and creative was *the very last thing*.[86,87] This capacity to make use of prosthetic devices during the archiving process to protect that which is absolutely essential to the self, leads me to question the significance of the dictaphone, on which this archive was recorded.

When I was preparing my proposed fieldwork for ethical approval, I had, at first, assumed that I would be able to record my sessions with all participants using my mobile telephone. However, I was told that this would not be possible, and that I should use a dictaphone instead. This was so that I could safely upload the anonymous sound files to a shared drive, before deleting them from the device itself. The dictaphone I purchased was black and discreet with several small buttons and was no longer than 15 centimetres long. The participants were strangely fascinated by this curious, foreign object, and would often reach over to move it closer to them as they were talking, and one lady (Participant 8) even picked it up and held it like a microphone on one occasion. Whilst it is possible to suggest that this interest in the recording device can be linked to the way in which the recorded word promises a different kind of promise within the future space of the archive, it is the attraction that the memory loss archivers appeared to have towards the dictaphone for use as a prosthetic memory recording device which is of interest here.

Derrida writes:

> I asked myself what is the moment *proper* to the archive, if there is such a thing, the instant of archivization strictly speaking, which is not, and I will come back to this, so-called live or spontaneous memory (*mnēmē or anamnēsis*), but rather a certain hypomnesic and prosthetic experience of the technical substrate.[88]

Here, once again, Derrida frames the archiving process as a kind of memory loss in itself. However, for the memory loss archivers, the attraction to the dictaphone may perhaps indicate an understanding of the potential benefits of technological manipulation, in which they were, once again, attempting to make use of the prosthetic potential of their recorded voices to house and protect the absolute truth. What comes to light here is that, just as with the archive itself, whilst the technological recordings offer a promise of a place in a future space, they do not and *cannot* offer a promise of meaning as the meaning of the archive can only happen in the future space, and is at the mercy of the (potential but never guaranteed) future auditor, whoever that may be. However, what the recordings taken on the dictaphone *can* offer is a possibility of repetition of truth, which can happen in the future space, even after the owner of the recorded voice has died. The participants' attempts to manipulate the recording device by touching it or picking it up provide a visual representation of the tension that exists between the internal and external life of both the archive and the memory loss experience itself, and how the memory loss archiver may uncannily hope to 'keep living' through a prosthetic object, in which the truth can be concealed. Derrida writes:

> And with this *domestic outside*, that is to say also with the hypothesis of an *internal* substrate, surface, or space without which there is neither consignation, registration, impression nor suppression, censorship, repression, it prepares the idea of a psychic archive distinct from spontaneous memory, of a *hypomnēsis* distinct from *mnēmē*, and from *anamnēsis*: the institution, in sum, of a *prosthesis of the inside*.[89]

In other words, *despite* their memory loss, when gathering this archive, the participants were able to use the recording device to move what was *absolutely necessary* from the inside to the prosthetic outside, in an attempt to secure a place in the promised future space. There is more thinking to do here, particularly concerning the problematic reflexive nature of the archiving process, in which, rather than a way to 'keep living', a recorded repetition of thought might actually be a way to 'keep dying' after death, and also the way in which the recordings have moved from the recording device itself and now exist on what is known as a 'cloud', but this would need more words than I have available in these short pages. Instead, I must now turn to the significance of the third party in this strangest of archival processes; me.

My role during the data gathering process was to develop personalised tasks using the creative practices that I have available to me (predominantly writing and music making) in order to provide the participants with the best possible opportunity to share their experiences in a way that was favourable to them. This allowed me to collect meaningful data, which provided me with a unique and new insight into the memory loss experience, as was my aim. I had to act extremely quickly during my fieldwork, due to the issues of capacity to consent and the urgency that comes with working with people who are coming to the end of their lives. There were many factors that made this challenging, including the way in which people who are living with memory loss tire easily because of sensory overload, and I also had to work around other logistical factors such as visits from families or the local nurse, all of which were not possible to plan around and had to take priority over my fieldwork. This meant that I had to arrive each day with a set of pre-planned, personalised sessions, not knowing who I would be able to work with that day. In terms of my influence over the data, I was acutely aware of the impact that I was having when I was gathering the archival material, and I made every attempt to ensure that I worked flexibly, sensitively, and creatively, in order to gather the most useful and meaningful material, in line with the ethos of the IPA methodology. This approach has meant that, when attempting to place this archive within a literary genre, it might be thought of as a brain memoir. In *The Elusive Brain: Literary Experiments in the Age of Neuroscience*, Jason Tougaw writes, "Although the ostensible subject of brain memoirs is the writer's particular subjective experience of an illness, difference, disorder, or injury, very often these memoirs become vehicles for large questions about the relationship between brain and self" and he goes on to say that brain memoirists use narrative, "to approximate the impossible: the revelation of another person's conscious experience."[90,91,92] In other words, in collecting narrative data in order to better understand the memory loss experience, I have created an archive which can be defined as a brain memoir, which, therefore, names me as a *brain memoirist*. Tougaw then comments that:

> brain memorists simulate their phenomenologies in language and narrative, inviting readers to imagine the experience. In the process, they involve readers in a kind of experiment in developing a metacognitive awareness about relations between the mind styles they've brought to the text and those the text simulates. Where many traditional memoirs take selfhood for granted, brain memoirs investigate how mind, brain, body and culture interact to create or perform selfhood, and that investigation has social, scientific, and philosophical implications. In fact, recent brain memoirs may have a thing or two to teach neuroscientists about the self, and they certainly have quite a bit to teach the rest of us about the functional and theoretical promises and limits of current brain research.[93]

Here, Tougaw acknowledges the importance of studies that use narrative data to understand and de-code different experiences. What he does not mention, however, is the *impact* that the memoirist has upon the data that is collected.

Due to the nature of the data-gathering process in IPA research studies, the IPA researcher must be aware of their own influence over the data that they have gathered and keep this in mind at the point of analysis. As such, the IPA framework acknowledges the role of the researcher, not just at the stage of data collection but also at the time of analytic interpretation. There are many places within the archive where my presence has a direct impact. The sound of my voice features heavily in all of the recordings, my words are written in the transcriptions of the interviews, and the tasks and games that I played with the participants were all devised by me. It is also possible to see how the increased familiarity that the participants felt towards me over time affected the data. This was due to the uncanny half-recognition that people who are living with memory loss feel when they see someone that they recognise but do not remember why. This increased sense of strange familiarity (caused, as I have postulated before, by the uncanniness of the memory loss experience) had an impact on all of the participants that were able to complete more than one session (you will remember this caused a particular problem with Participant 4 who knew she did not like talking to me but did not know why until I mentioned music to her) and seemed, in some respects, to dilute the urgency of the archival impulse that is very recognisable in all of the first sessions, and seems to diminish in all sessions with all participants as they progress.

Derrida suggests that the role of the archivist is one that inevitably adds to the archive itself, in all archival processes; "One will never be able to objectivize it with no remainder. The archivist produces more archive, and that is why the archive is never closed. It opens out of the future." I am reminded here of Kelman's, "No matter the outcome I would discover something of it, more of it, and here it is of the future."[94] While I would agree that this is the case, I would argue that the role of the archivist is even more predominant in research that follows an IPA research methodology such as this, because of the way in which the methodology relies on the role of the archivist to generate the archival material.[95] This means that the reflexive nature of the archival process is intensified by the IPA process, which makes the relationship between the archive and the future even more problematic. Derrida writes:

> the archive, as printing, writing, prosthesis, or hypmomnesic technique in general is not only the place for stocking and for conserving an archivable content *of the past* which would exist in any case, such as, without the archive, one still believes it was or will have been. No, the technical structure of the *archiving* archive also determines the structure of the *archivable* content even in its very coming into existence and in its relationship to the future.[96]

As with all archives, the structure of the archival content in this particular archive is influenced by many things, including (as previously discussed) the relationship between the two archivers, the recording device, and the 'home' in which the archive was gathered. However, what is different about this archive is that, in making use of tools of adaptation, such as prosthesis, in order to adapt to the memory loss experience, the memory loss archiver creates an archive which has an increased plasticity than that of an archive which does not include an archiver who is living with memory loss.

In *What Should We Do With Our Brain?,* Catherine Malabou writes:[97]

> plasticity directly contradicts rigidity. It is its exact antonym. In ordinary speech, it designates suppleness, a faculty for adaptation, the ability to evolve. According to its etymology – from the Greek *plassein,* to mold – the word *plasticity* has two basic senses: it means at once the capacity to *receive form* (clay is called "plastic," for example) and the capacity to *give form* (as in the plastic arts or in plastic surgery).[98]

In this sense, and in line with my reading of Derrida thus far, it is possible to suggest that all archives can be considered to be plastic, particularly when Malabou goes on to say, "But it must be remarked that plasticity is also the capability to annihilate the very form it is able to receive or create."[99] Tougaw writes, "Malabou emphasizes the fact that the brain works through representation, registering and representing stimuli in the world through neural connections. The brain's plasticity, its capacity to change, imbricates its *representation* of the world with that world" and whilst this may be the case for all brains, the memory loss brain appears to use plasticity in a slightly different way.[100]

In *What I wish people knew about dementia, from someone who knows*, Mitchell mentions a study that highlighted the way in which people living with memory loss were able to 'hold on' to the memories that defined their sense of self.[101] She writes:

> In Marie Mills's 1997 study, one man with advanced dementia was able to talk in great detail about his time as a prisoner of war. Researchers noted the importance of this: 'They were the type of memories which … 'live long in the memory of the mind,' for they tended to be significantly concerned with the individual physical and psychological survival of the self. The intensity of effort to survive during his time as a prisoner of war may have created these durable memories which appeared to withstand the onslaught of dementia, almost until the end … His stories allowed him to be readily seen as a 'whole' person. This gave him a sense of narrative identity and underlines the importance of the maintenance of narrative during this illness.[102]

I saw this many times during the course of my fieldwork, and even in cases where these narrative memories had been suppressed, they were liberated by the sound world of the nursing home environment, as I have previously postulated. However, what Mills does not mention, is what happens to these important, identity-defining memories, in cases when the memory loss state does not allow for them to be articulated freely. It would be easy to suggest that, when this becomes the case in the later phases of the memory loss experience, the identity of the person is then lost. However, this is where I have found the memory loss archiver to *challenge* the equation of "self = memory" and "loss of memory = loss of self," because I have found that the memories are *not* lost, and, therefore, neither is the identity of the person who is living with memory loss.[103] On the contrary, what I have found to happen is that people who are living with memory loss are able to plasticly adapt to their memory loss state, and they do this via a manipulation of the prosthetic. This means that people who are living with memory loss are able to show what is absolutely necessary, or the truth, if the person who is listening is able to read through and into their use of the prosthetic. The implication of this, in terms of the archive, is that, although all archives can be considered to be plastic, this particular archive has an *increased* plasticity, due to the plasticity of the memory loss experience itself, which is created by the way in which the participants were able to adapt to the later stages of the memory loss experience via a manipulation of the prosthetic. This is evident in the way in which the memory loss archiver has demonstrated an ability to give form and receive form (by being able to reveal a combination of suppressed and repressed feelings) whilst also adapting to the experience by making use of the prosthetic, before reaching a destructive end in the form of fatal repetition. As such, my reading of Derrida and Malabou in this context means that it is possible to look upon this archive as a kind of plastic art making, in which the participants and I are engaged in an ongoing creative process which is malleable, shape-shifting, and supple that may or may not exist in the here/there, what/where, maybe/maybe not archive in the within/without of the unpromisable future space.

The memory loss brain is an intelligent brain that sometimes borders on the magical. It is capable of adapting, changing, and learning so that the identity of the person it inhabits may survive. There is never a loss of self; the self continues to exist within the truth, which a person living with memory loss is able to show, right up until the very last thing, whatever that may be. This archive shows that, "self = memory" and "loss of memory = loss of self"[104], is, in fact, not the case, and whilst there are destructive drives at play within the memory loss experience (magnified here by placing these stories within an archive; a destructive force in itself), the material that I have gathered suggests that people living with memory loss are able to hold onto the self until the very last moment. This ability to adapt to an experience which is uncannily splitting and doubling, whilst also balancing (and making use of) the tension that exists between the desire to live and the desire to die, is both remarkable, and remarkably human. Or, to return to Smith:

> It's the act of making it up, from the combination of what we've got and what we haven't, that makes the human, makes the art, makes this transformation possible, like it's the eye engaged in the creative act, in union with a kind of not seeing.[105]

However, whilst I have found that people living with memory loss are able to adapt to the memory loss experience, the question remains of how people who are *not* living with memory loss might also adapt to the experience too, and at this moment, I would like to begin to offer a new perspective.

Different, not less

> When people think of dementia, they immediately associate it with memory. Few people realise, for example, just how it changes our relationships with our senses, our emotions, our communication. Few people understand the importance of a good environment – both inside and out – after a dementia diagnosis, and the small changes that make a big difference.[106]
>
> – *Wendy Mitchell, What I wish people knew about dementia, from someone who knows*

At the beginning of this book, I promised to offer, not only a new and valuable insight into the memory loss experience but also a fresh perspective and new approach to how we might think about memory loss. It is at this point that I would like to begin to offer that new perspective, but first I must explain why. I have worked as a teacher of music and English to young people between the ages of 11 and 18 since 2009, and, in many respects, my career has been varied. Among other things, I have taught music in a very large state school in greater London, I have directed large choirs, I have taught the flute, and I have taught English to children with profound physical and mental illnesses who were too unwell to attend school. However, whilst these roles have demanded a range of approaches, the ethos of my teaching has always been the same; I believe that it is my responsibility to understand (as well as I can) the lived experiences of my students and then use that information to adapt my practice to ensure that they can learn well and happily, and I have gathered this archive using the same ethos. Tougaw writes:

> the other people in the subjects' social spheres – physicians, caretakers, loved ones – must learn to adapt. They must create an environment that enables and encourages the expression and agency that emerge from a particular person's neurological eccentricities – what many now may call *neurodivergence*.[107]

In other words, when trying to understand how a neurological condition affects a particular person's lived experience, it is necessary for the person that is seeking that information (in this case, me) to adapt their practice accordingly so that the person is able to express themselves in a way that suits them, as is the case with studies such as this that follow an IPA methodology, and as I have done during this data gathering process. In doing this, I have come to learn that, in order to understand the memory loss experience, it is helpful to think of the memory loss state as a kind of neurodivergence.

On a definition of neurodivergence, the Oxford English Dictionary offers:

1 "Divergence in mental or neurological functioning from what is considered typical or normal, esp. where this falls on the autism spectrum; the state or quality of being neurodivergent."[108]

And, whilst Merriam-Webster does not currently offer a definition of neurodivergence, it has the following as a definition of *neurodiversity*:

1 "Individual differences in brain functioning regarded as normal variations within the human population.
2 The concept that differences in brain functioning within the human population are normal and that brain functioning that is not neurotypical should not be stigmatized.
3 The inclusion in a group, organisation, etc. of people of different types of brain functioning."[109]

Using these definitions, it is possible to suggest that the data that I have collected during this process indicates that the memory loss experience falls into the category of neurodivergence (or neurodiversity), particularly when considering the similarities between the memory loss experience and other conditions which are considered to be neurodivergent, such as autism. These similarities are plenty, and the most obvious examples from this research include sensory processing difficulties, a tendency and ability to 'mask' (using 'stock' answers and phrases, distraction techniques, and prosthetic words), and a sensitivity to certain sounds.

The reason this is a useful way to think about the memory loss experience is that it helps to de-catastrophise a memory loss diagnosis whilst demonstrating that people living with memory loss are able to adapt to their new experience, thus encouraging a fresh perspective in which the memory loss experience can be understood. This idea is echoed by several other researchers, including in the work of neurodivergent researcher, Linda Örulv.

Örulv is a neurodiverse communication ethnographer within the field of dementia studies who, like me, works to de-catastrophise a memory loss diagnosis by using qualitative research methodologies to shed further light on the memory loss experience. Of her work, she writes, "As a contrast to the 'personal tragedy' that often accompanies a one-sidedly medical model for understanding the condition(s), I have emphasised how residents in dementia residential care actively used their remaining linguistic and cognitive resources to make sense of their situations, their surroundings and their lives."[110] What is of interest here is that the similarity in our research approaches has led to a similar theory; that it is possible to think of the memory loss experience as a kind of neurodiversity. Örulv acknowledges that the difficulty with this theory is the differences between dementia and other neurodiverse diagnoses with, "While dementia sets in as a disruption to the functioning that is already in place, autism is often likened to functioning from a different 'operative system' altogether and is described by self-advocates as something that is deeply integrated into the very core of one's personality."[111] However, Örulv maintains that a neurodiverse lens is a helpful tool when thinking about and designing care and therapeutic interventions for people who are living with memory loss, and, for this, she turns to Chapman;

> Chapman (2020b, p.219) proposes that neurodiversity is 'more of an epistemically useful concept than anything else' insofar as it 'helps us imagine the world differently to how it currently is.' He further suggests that 'by adopting a neurodiversity perspective, we can alter actual relations; all the way from how we empathize with neurological others on a personal level, to how we design scientific experiments or public spaces' (p.220), something that may eventually change our shared world for the better.[112]

In other words, understanding the memory loss state as a kind of neurodiversity allows for the possibility for adaptations to thinking and practice, thus making an inclusive approach to the way in which we react to, treat, and think about a memory loss diagnosis a possibility. This perspective is one that I adopted several years ago following a visit to my late grandfather in June 2018. I wrote the following in my diary that evening:

"Visited PP tonight. It was still light when I arrived but the whole home felt really dark and quiet on the inside, and there was that strange glow in his room that's sometimes there in the evenings that makes it look purple. I still can't work out where it comes from because it vanishes when you lift the net curtains. Maybe it's the moon? Or the sun? Or both? It's a strange light because it feels like it hits you at hip

height, rather than coming from above. Anyway, he was in bed and half asleep, but he seemed quite pleased when I arrived. I probably should have just sat there and not said anything, but the woman in the opposite room kept calling for help, and I was trying to talk over her so that she didn't disturb him - he looked like he needed some peace and quiet. I was exhausted (long day, long story) and couldn't think of much to say, so I ended up telling him about mum's new curtains. I forgot myself and stupidly called her mum, at which point he looked at me in horror and said, "Mum? My wife? I thought she was dead?" Then I had to explain (again) that; "My mum is your daughter and yes your wife is dead and she's been dead for years about thirteen now and you have a new partner now who you've also been with for years and you've been on lots of cruises and look that's her in the photograph and yes she does still visit she came today because I saw her name in the signing in book but she won't be up tomorrow because tomorrow is Saturday and that's when she does her hair and yes mum comes too and mum wrote on the whiteboard by the door (that you can't see but it's over there) that she has bought you a new shirt from Marks and Spencer but it hasn't arrived yet but she will bring it up as soon as it arrives in the post and yes it's being posted to her house instead of here because things sometimes get lost when they get posted here don't they like the slippers did that time but don't worry about it because she got you another pair look they're by my feet on the floor they're huge I've never known anyone to have such big feet as you I can still fit both of mine into one of these look! ooh they're lovely and soft but they're hot in this weather and mum managed to find the exact shirt that you wanted with the soft collar which will look nice on y(our) birthday and I think she said that it's blue and stripey but not big stripes no but very thin stripes I think they're white the stripes not the shirt the shirt is blue I think I think mum said it's navy but I'm not sure she hasn't written that on the whiteboard so I don't know and do you want a cup of tea it's a bit late now isn't it but I can make you one in the kitchen if you want one because I don't think the lady will come around again until the morning now." And then his eyes rolled into the back of his head and he fell into a lifeless sleep, so I gave him a kiss and left. I tried to write something on the whiteboard, but I didn't know what to write, so I put the pen lid back on and left.

I was so cross with myself all the way home. It's a tiny, three letter word, but every time I say mum it completely throws him, and I've had to tell him that his wife is dead so many times now, and every time it's as though he's being told for the first time. It's devastating. I try so hard not to say it but it's so difficult. I'm going to try really hard not to do it again. I've decided that I'm not taking photos up anymore either, and I'm not going to buy anything else that promises to magically bring his memory back (a talking photo album full of pictures of dead people? What was I thinking?) and I'm just going to take him as I find him each time, and try to talk about things that are happening now, rather than a past that he can't remember or a future that we do not have. If I stop focusing on his memory (or lack of it) and concentrate on trying to understand how he is feeling, then maybe this will be a bit less frightening. I feel a bit better now, but I wish I had written on the whiteboard when I left tonight. He won't know that I was there."

After that moment, my relationship with my grandfather changed completely. It is not easy to describe, and, in many ways, words escape me here, not because writing about it makes me feel sad, but rather because my relationship with him had always felt like something other, or something else, as all relationships do with the people that we give over our thoughts to and they to us, as we sit beside them, during life and also during death. If I am to bring words to what it felt like I would say that it felt like a friendship that was free from context or agenda. We sat together for many hours in Room Number 247 (usually with him in the bed and me on the chair, fiddling with his slippers on the floor with my feet), and we would talk about the seasons, or animals, or the dreams that we had had. Sometimes he would tell me about the other person in the room (who I was too blind to see) and I would listen carefully as he described who they were, what they looked like, and what they were doing. On one occasion, with his eyes scrunched closed, he told me that he was frightened because he didn't want to hurt himself or get into trouble. I asked him what he could see, and he described the kitchen in the home that he had lived in as a young boy – the countertops were head height, and his small hands could just about reach up to steal some cake that had been left on the side. His stories in those moments taught me so much about his life. In fact, I learned far more than I ever did by trying to jog his memory as I did in the months that followed his diagnosis. I have already mentioned how beautiful his storytelling became during his last months; each fragment of precious information would come back again and again, so gently but with absolute purpose, and often when he was in a hypnogogic state. Later on, when his storytelling had reached its end ("words make me sick") he would look at me with gentle and familiar eyes when I entered the room that would show me that he knew me and that he was pleased that I was there. For my grandfather, acknowledging his family (who he had always described as his pride and joy) and showing us that he knew who we were in order to save our sadness, was *the very last thing.*

Making the decision to change my perspective in June of 2018, thawed all of the fear I had about my grandfather losing his memory, and it allowed both of us to spend many contended hours together until his death in February of 2019. To put it simply, we adapted to one another; he with his beautiful, clever, memory-loss brain, and me with my changed perspective, and we met somewhere in the middle. Just as the participants did in this study, my grandfather was able to use the prosthetic (which for him, took the form of repetitive folk tales and ghost stories) in order to continue to communicate and keep living, right up until the very last moment. This meant that we could happily relax into the safety of each other's company, which allowed us to form new memories and connect with one another, even when we were doing not very much at all. I did not know it at the time, but, in the end, in deciding to adapt to his memory loss state, and moving the needle of my focus from his memory loss to trying to understand his experience and learn from it, I gifted us both eight precious months of time together which we would not have otherwise had.

The need for a change of perspective and an adaptation of approach when trying to understand the memory loss experience creeps in among analysists from the 1990s onwards, and interestingly, and, perhaps, surprisingly, even Oliver Sacks' approach to analysing his patients changed as he approached the end of his career. Tougaw cites the following from the preface of Sacks' text from 1996, *An Anthropologist on Mars*:

> In earlier books I wrote of the 'preservation' of self, and (more rarely) of the 'loss' of self, in neurological disorders. I have come to think these terms too simple – and that there is neither loss nor preservation of identity in such situations, but, rather, its adaptation, even its transmutation, given a radically altered brain and 'reality'.[113]

In adopting (what I would argue to be) a more inclusive and open-minded approach to his subjects, Sacks was able to begin to see past the unhelpful narrative of his previous work and discover the brain's ability to adapt to its changing or changed status. Like Sacks, I also saw this 'adaptation' and 'transmutation' many times during this process, particularly in the use of the prosthetic or 'stock' answers that I saw in all participants, and I have previously used Malabou's ideas about artistic plasticity to illustrate this. However, in this next moment, I would like to look at Malabou's theories alongside theories of *neuro*plasticity, in an attempt to offer a new perspective of the memory loss experience, whilst also positioning the outcomes of this research within the field of the medical humanities.

For a definition of neuroplasticity, the Oxford English Dictionary has:

1 "The ability of the nervous system to form and reorganize connections and pathways, as during development and learning or following injury."[114]

And Merriam-Webster has it as:

1 "The capacity for continuous alteration of the neural pathways and synapses of the living brain and nervous system in response to experience or injury."[115]

And Mitchell writes:

> We often talk about neuroplasticity, where our brain may be damaged in one place but uses another route to enable us to do or remember things. If the motorway is closed, we use the B roads, and that's what our brain does too, even in someone with dementia.[116]

This idea that the brain is polymorphic, particularly in circumstances where it has experienced distress in some form, has been illustrated many times by the participants who were living with memory loss during this process, and each participant demonstrated an ability to adapt to their memory loss experience in order to protect their identity. However, it is possible to suggest that this ability to adapt goes beyond the capability to protect what is already there, and demonstrates an ability to learn *new* things. Malabou writes, "The idea of cellular renewal, repair, and resourcefulness as auxiliaries of synaptic plasticity brings to light the power of *healing* – treatment, scarring, compensation, regeneration, and the capacity of the brain to build natural prosthesis."[117] This idea of what Malabou calls a "natural prosthesis" is key to the findings of this investigation, as it places the prosthetic within the future space, along with the archive itself.[118] It also opens up the possibility for a discussion around the healing qualities of a verbal archiving process (such as this one), due to the fact that the prosthetic devices that the participants used were all language based. Malabou continues:

> The plastic art of the brain gives birth to a statue capable of self-repair. We know full well that the functioning of the brain can be disturbed by numerous pathological causes, the best-known being cranial trauma, strokes, encephalitis, and neurodivergence disorders (Parkinson's, Alzheimer's). But the nervous system always demonstrates plasticity after such handicaps or lesions, whether or not these efforts are crowned with success: the affected structures or functions try to modify themselves so as to compensate for the new deficit or form a new and abnormal organizational schema that restores normalcy.[119]

This potential for the memory loss brain, not only to repair itself but to learn new things, is key to the ethos of this study for two reasons. Firstly, it places the person who is living with memory loss in the future space, which is in direct contrast to the way in which we are conditioned to think about the memory loss experience, whilst also encouraging a new and helpful shift in perspective in which the memory loss brain could be seen to have *value*. Secondly, it opens up the possibility for a shift in the way in which we treat people who are living with memory loss; music therapy, for example, could change its aim from trying to use music to trigger memories (which, as I have postulated many times, is often an unkind practice) and focus instead on teaching new and enjoyable skills, and nursing homes could stop surrounding people with strange and frightening artefacts from the past and instead introduce people to new things. And whilst it is possible to suggest that neurotypical brains also make use of plasticity, looking at plasticity through a lens of neurodivergence and brain trauma illuminates the brilliance of the memory loss brain, whilst also shedding further light on the theory of plasticity itself. Malabou continues:

> Another example is what happens at the onset of Alzheimer's disease. The encroaching amnesia is compensated for in part by a capacity to recuperate stored information. The deactivation of certain regions (the region of the hippocampus), is balanced by a metabolic activation of other regions (the frontal regions). Thus after certain circuits are affected, there is a modification in strategies for handling information, a modification that again attests to the functional plasticity of the brain.[120]

This is an idea that Malabou expands upon in her later text, *The New Wounded: From Neurosis to Brain Damage,* in which she focuses her attention on people who experience psychic wounds caused by cerebral lesions such as Alzheimer's disease.[121] She begins by explaining that her motivation for writing the books was, "a belated reaction to the ordeal of depersonalization to which my grandmother was subjected as Alzheimer's disease operated upon her."[122] Malabou's personal relationship with the memory loss experience is of obvious interest here, and, she too, begins the text with some personal reflections and hypotheses developed during her grandmother's time with dementia. She writes:

> Indeed, this was not a diminished person in front of me, the same woman weaker than she used to be, lessened, spoiled. No, this was a stranger who didn't recognize me, who didn't recognize herself because she had undoubtedly never met her before. Behind the familiar halo of hair, the tone of her voice, the blue of her eyes: the absolutely incontestable presence of *someone else.*[123]

In taking this initial standpoint, Malabou suggests that a memory loss state might be thought of as a catastrophic end to psychic life in which the person is replaced by another being. She goes on to write, "A person with Alzheimer's disease, for example, is not – or not only – someone who has 'changed' or been 'modified', but rather *a subject who has become someone else.*"[124] She then begins to explore what this hypothesis might mean for her existing theories of neuroplasticity, by staging a confrontation between the ideas of neurology and psychoanalysis.

Initially, Malabou postulates that a memory loss state might challenge Freud's idea of the death drive, by being a state that is entered into following a death of the 'self' which, in itself, might be thought of as a kind of metamorphic process towards death that is devoid of desire and psychic life. She asks the question, "Could it be that there is a type of suffering that creates a new identity, the unknown identity of an unknown person who suffers? Could it be that cerebral suffering is precisely such suffering?" and she refers to this idea again towards the end of the text, in which she refers to a memory loss state as a, "type of transformation into death, this survival without sublation."[125,126] However, she challenges this idea when she looks at the memory loss state from a perspective of 'destructive' or 'postlesional' plasticity.

On destructive and postlesional plasticity, Malabou writes, "There is postlesional plasticity that is not the plasticity of reconstruction but the default formation of a new identity with loss as its premise" and she goes on to say that, "Lesional plasticity thus reveals a strange sculptural power that produces form through the annihilation of form."[127,128] This idea of the memory loss brain's ability to rebuild and reconstruct, not just in spite of, but *because of* the way in which it continuously annihilates itself, is in keeping with the findings of this study, in that it supports the idea that the memory loss brain is capable of learning new things, whilst protecting the identity of the person that it inhabits as they exist, not as a new person or as *someone else*, but as an alternate way of being, because, as Malabou has it, "the disruption of cerebral auto-affection does not put an end to psychic life."[129]

Knowing that the memory loss brain is capable of using destructive or postlesional plasticity to adapt to its changing status is, of course, helpful when trying to understand the memory loss experience, and I have collected many examples of this being the case during this process. This ability to constantly break down and rebuild is particularly impressive when considering the way that the memory loss status seems to continually change through a reflexive process of doubling and splitting. However, during the later phases of the memory loss experience, the ability to adapt can become more challenging, which is why it is necessary for the people that surround those living with memory loss to understand the experience, and adapt their perspective and practices accordingly.

During our second interview, Mitchell said:[130]

"***Sam:*** The first one is actually about the dementia experience as a whole. One of the things I'm trying to do is to understand how it feels to have dementia. In the media, and in society, all of the focus is on memory loss, and I'm learning that it's so much more than that. And I was just wondering if you would be able to, in your own words, tell me how dementia feels to you?

Wendy: This is the most asked question I get asked. So, I can probably do my talk off by heart. Let's see. Imagine the brain is a string of fairy lights, with each fairy light representing a different function of the brain. But different fairy lights flicker and fail for each of us. So that's why some people can cook, and I can't. That's why they feel hunger, but I don't. That's why I can type, and others can't. So, I can type words quicker than I can think and speak them, because that part, that light bulb, hasn't extinguished. But different light bulbs flicker and fail for all of us. So, when the light bulb fails altogether, that's when that specific ability has been taken away for good, and that's why I concentrate on the light bulbs that still work. I don't dwell on the ones that are extinguished, because I can't bring them back again. I just concentrate on what I can do, not what I can't. Does that help?"[131]

Here, Mitchell explains how the memory loss experience feels to her, in her current phase of the experience, and she uses the analogy of switching fairy lights off to explain how she adapts to her changing brain. However, the reason she recites this speech at many of her talks during her outreach work is because she believes that it is important for people who are not living with memory loss to understand the memory loss experience. She does this to educate them, and to inform the development of future practice, because she believes that, in order for the memory loss experience to become a liveable condition, it is necessary for those who are not living with memory loss to attempt to understand the condition, and to adapt to it, by making "the small changes that make a big difference."[132] I would argue that by thinking of the memory loss experience as a kind of neurodiversity, and also by taking into account the brain's ability, not only to adapt to the experience but to learn new things, it is possible to de-catastrophise a memory loss diagnosis in a way that makes a kind and inclusive space for people who are living with memory loss within our culture.

My primary aim when writing this chapter was to offer a new insight into the memory loss experience. My hope is that, by looking at the data that I have gathered in the context of the uncanny, the nursing home environment, the death drive, archival impulses, prosthetic manipulation, artistic plasticity, and neuroplasticity, I have made a small and useful step towards the demystification of the memory loss experience. The participants in this study have demonstrated not only how complicated the memory loss experience is, but how clever the memory loss brain is at adapting to the experience whilst also being able to learn new things. I hope that, in offering this new understanding of the way in which the memory loss brain operates, I have opened up the possibility for a change in perspective, which could encourage a more inclusive approach to thought, theory, and practice, and is in line with the ethos of this research; that an identity changed by memory loss is different, not less.

Notes

1 Royle, N. (2003) *The Uncanny.* Manchester: Manchester University Press. p. 6.
2 Freud, S. (1919) 'The Uncanny,' in Strachey, A. (1985), in *Pelican Freud Library, vol.14* Harmondsworth: Penguin, pp 339–376.
3 Freud, S. (1919) P370.
4 Freud, S. (1919) P340.
5 Royle, N. (2003) *The Uncanny.* Manchester: Manchester University Press.
6 Royle, N. (2003) P2.
7 Royle, N. (2003) P6.
8 Schlipphacke, H. (2015) 'The Place and Time of the Uncanny', in *Pacific Coast Philology*. Penn State University Press, p 165.
9 Davis Basting, A. (2009) *Forget Memory.* The John Hopkins University Press: Baltimore. P24.
10 Mitchell, W. (2019) *Somebody I Used to Know.* London: Bloomsbury Publishing. P252.
11 Mitchell, W. (2019) P254.
12 Zeller, F. (2015) *The Mother and the Father.* (Trans. From French by C. Hampton). London: Faber & Faber.
13 See Chapter 2 PP 9–28.
14 Mitchell, W (2022) *Which me am I today?* [online] Available at: https://whichmeamitoday.wordpress.com/blog/ [Accessed: May 9th, 2022]
15 Mitchell, W. (2019)
16 Appendix Y. www.routledge.com/9781041072652
17 Carrington, L. with Smith, A. (2005) *The Hearing Trumpet.* London: Penguin Classics. P13.
18 Royle, N. (2003) P1.
19 Royle, N. (2003) P1.
20 Appendix K. www.routledge.com/9781041072652
21 Appendix K. www.routledge.com/9781041072652
22 Appendix CC. www.routledge.com/9781041072652
23 Appendix CC. www.routledge.com/9781041072652

24 Appendix K. www.routledge.com/9781041072652
25 Royle, N. (2003) P6.
26 Appendix CC. www.routledge.com/9781041072652
27 Royle, N. (2003) P2.
28 Shanklin, W. (1951) *Jezebel* (song). Columbia.
29 Appendix CC. www.routledge.com/9781041072652
30 Appendix M. www.routledge.com/9781041072652
31 Royle, N. (2003) P5.
32 Appendix CC. www.routledge.com/9781041072652
33 Shanklin, W. (1951) *Jezebel* (song). Columbia.
34 Freud, S. (1920) 'Beyond the pleasure principle', in Phillips, A. (2006) *The Penguin Freud reader.* London: Penguin, pp 132–195.
35 Freud, S. (1920) P166.
36 Freud, S. (1920) P140.
37 Freud, S. (1919)
38 Freud, S. (1920) P185.
39 Carrington, L. with Smith, A. (2005) P13.
40 Mitchell, W. (2023) *One Last Thing: How to live with the end in mind.* London: Bloomsbury Publishing.
41 Mitchell, W. (2023) PP133–137.
42 Mitchell, W. (2023) P136.
43 Carrington, L. with Smith, A. (2005) P13.
44 Oxford English Dictionary. (2023) *Archive, n., sense 3* [online] Available at: https://www.oed.com/dictionary/archive_n?tab=meaning_and_use [Accessed: November the 13th, 2023]
45 Merriam-Webster. (2023) *Archive* [online] Available at: https://www.merriam-webster.com/dictionary/archive?src=search-dict-box [Accessed: November 13th, 2023]
46 Derrida, J. (1996) *Archive Fever: A Freudian Impression.* (Trans. From French by E. Prenowitz), Chicago and London: The University of Chicago Press.
47 Derrida, J. (1996) P1.
48 Derrida, J. (1996) P2.
49 Derrida, J. (1996) P29.
50 Derrida, J. (1996) P36.
51 Derrida, J. (1996) P36.
52 Derrida, J. (1996) PP2–3.
53 Coetzee, J.M. (2017) P219.
54 Derrida, J. (1996) P29.
55 Derrida, J. (1996) P29.
56 Derrida, J. (1996) PP29–30.
57 Derrida, J. (1996) P30.
58 Appendix DD. www.routledge.com/9781041072652 and Appendix EE. www.routledge.com/9781041072652
59 Freud, S. (1919) p 370.
60 Derrida, J. (1996) P28.
61 Derrida, J. (1996) P28.
62 Appendix L. www.routledge.com/9781041072652
63 Appendix Q. www.routledge.com/9781041072652
64 See Chapter 3, Case Study 4, The Dying Artist. PP78–80.
65 Appendix Y. www.routledge.com/9781041072652
66 Appendix W. www.routledge.com/9781041072652
67 Shanklin, W. (1951)
68 See Chapter 3, Case Study 2, Participant 4. PP45–61.

69 See Chapter 3, See Case Study 2, Participant 4. PP45–61.
70 Freud, S. (1920) P140.
71 Appendix R. www.routledge.com/9781041072652
72 Derrida, J. (1996) P68.
73 Freud, S. (1920) P185.
74 Derrida, J. (1996) P10.
75 Derrida, J. (1996) P11.
76 Derrida, J. (1996) P12.
77 Davis Basting, A. (2009) P24.
78 Appendix Z.
79 See Chapter 3, Case Study 5, Participant 6. PP82–98.
80 Derrida, J. (1996) P87.
81 See Chapter 3, Case Study 5, Participant 6. PP82–98.
82 Derrida, J. (1996) P88.
83 Derrida, J. (1996) P88.
84 See Chapter 3, Case Study 5, Participant 6. PP82–98.
85 Derrida, J. (1996) P12.
86 See Chapter 3, Case Study 5, Participant 6. PP82–98.
87 See Chapter 3, Case Study 4, The Dying Artist. PP78–80.
88 Derrida, J. (1996) P25.
89 Derrida, J. (1996) P19.
90 Tougaw, J. (2018) *The Elusive Brain: Literary Experiments in the Age of Neuroscience.* United States of America: Yale University Press.
91 Tougaw, J. (2018) P75.
92 Tougaw, J. (2018) P75.
93 Tougaw, J. (2018) P76.
94 Kelman, J. (2002) P13.
95 Derrida, J. (1996) P68.
96 Derrida, J. (1996) P17.
97 Malabou, C. (2008) *What Should We Do with Our Brain?* New York: Fordham University Press.
98 Malabou, C. (2008) P5.
99 Malabou, C. (2008) P5.
100 Tougaw, J. (2018) P19.
101 Mitchell, W. (2022) *What I Wish People Knew about Dementia, from Someone Who Knows.* London: Bloomsbury Publishing.
102 Mitchell, W. (2022) P203.
103 Davis Basting, A. (2009) P24.
104 Davis Basting, A. (2009) P24.
105 Smith, A. (2013) P25.
106 Mitchell, W. (2022) P3.
107 Tougaw, J. (2018) P42.
108 Oxford English Dictionary. (2023) *Neurodivergence, n.* [online] Available at: https://www.oed.com/dictionary/neurodivergence_n?tab=meaning_and_use [Accessed: November 28, 2023]
109 Merriam-Webster. (2023) *Neurodiversity* [online] Available at: https://www.merriam-webster.com/dictionary/neurodiversity [Accessed: November 28th, 2023]
110 Örulv, L. (2023) 'Neurodiversity and Dementia: Pitfalls, Possibilities and Some Personal Notes', in Sandberg, L. J. and Ward, R. (eds.) *Critical Dementia Studies: An introduction*. New York: Taylor and Francis, p. 247
111 Örulv, L. (2023) p.250
112 Örulv, L. (2023) p. 255

113 Tougaw, J. (2018) PP41–42.
114 Oxford English Dictionary (2023) *Neuroplasticity, n.* [online] Available at: https://www.oed.com/dictionary/neuroplasticity_n?tab=meaning_and_use [Accessed: December 4th, 2023]
115 Merriam-Webster. (2023) *Plasticity, sense 3.* [online] Available at: *https://www.merriam-webster.com/dictionary/plasticity* [Accessed: December 4th, 2023]
116 Mitchell, W. (2022) PP154–155.
117 Malabou, C. (2008) P27.
118 Malabou, C. (2008) P27.
119 Malabou, C. (2008) PP27–28.
120 Malabou, C. (2008) PP28–29.
121 Malabou, C. (2012) *The New Wounded: From Neurosis to Brain Damage* (Trans. From French by S. Miller) New York: Fordham University Press.
122 Malabou, C. (2012) Pxi.
123 Malabou, C. (2012) Pxi.
124 Malabou, C. (2012) P15.
125 Malabou, C. (2012) Pxii.
126 Malabou, C. (2012) P213.
127 Malabou, C. (2012) P48.
128 Malabou, C. (2012) P49.
129 Malabou, C. (2012) P48.
130 Appendix CC. www.routledge.com/9781041072652
131 Appendix CC. www.routledge.com/9781041072652
132 Mitchell, W. (2022) P3.

Bibliography

Carrington, L. with Smith, A. (2005) *The Hearing Trumpet*. London: Penguin Classics.
Coetzee, J.M. (2017) *The Schooldays of Jesus*. London: Vintage.
Davis Basting, A. (2009) *Forget Memory*. Baltimore: The John Hopkins University Press.
Derrida, J. (1996) *Archive Fever: A Freudian Impression*. (Trans. From French by E. Prenowitz), Chicago and London: The University of Chicago Press.
Freud, S. (1919) 'The Uncanny', in Strachey, A. (1985), in *Pelican Freud Library, vol.14* Harmondsworth: Penguin, pp. 339–76.
Freud, S. (1920) 'Beyond the Pleasure Principle', in Phillips, A. (2006) *The Penguin Freud Reader*. London: Penguin, pp. 132–195.
Kelman, J. (2002) *Translated Accounts*. London: Vintage.
Malabou, C. (2008) *What Should We Do with Our Brain?* New York: Fordham University Press.
Malabou, C. (2012) *The New Wounded: From Neurosis to Brain Damage* (Trans. From French by S. Miller) New York: Fordham University Press.
Mitchell, W. (2019) *Somebody I Used to Know*. London: Bloomsbury Publishing.
Mitchell, W (2022) *Which me am I today?* [online] Available at: https://whichmeamitoday.wordpress.com/blog/ [Accessed: May 9th, 2022]
Mitchell, W. (2022) *What I Wish People Knew about Dementia from Someone Who Knows*. London: Bloomsbury Publishing.
Mitchell, W. (2023) *One Last Thing: How to Live with the End in Mind*. London: Bloomsbury Publishing.
Örulv, L. (2023) 'Neurodiversity and Dementia: Pitfalls, Possibilities and Some Personal Notes', in Sandberg, L. J. and Ward, R. (eds.) *Critical Dementia Studies: An Introduction*, New York: Taylor and Francis, pp. 247–262.
Royle, N. (2003) *The Uncanny*. Manchester: Manchester University Press.

Schlipphacke, H. (2015) 'The Place and Time of the Uncanny', in *Pacific Coast Philology*. Penn State University Press, pp. 163–172.
Shanklin, W. (1951) *Jezebel* (song). Columbia.
Smith, A. (2013) *Artful*. UK: Penguin.
Tougaw, J. (2018) *The Elusive Brain: Literary Experiments in the Age of Neuroscience*. United States of America: Yale University Press.
Zeller, F. (2015) *The Mother and the Father*. (Trans. From French by C. Hampton), London: Faber & Faber.

Chapter 5

An alternate way of being and implications for future practice

The truth is the process of gathering, analysing, and discussing this set of data has been dizzyingly reflexive. Each time I have brought a thought or a theory to this curious archive, the archive has taught me more about the thought or the theory than the archive itself. This archive behaves (and misbehaves) very similarly to the memory loss brain, and if I had not been able to use musical composition as a research tool alongside my thinking, I am not sure whether I would have been able to make any sense out of it at all. This creative approach, combined with five case studies analysed in line with the interpretative phenomenological analysis methodology, and a discussion that is grounded in theories of psychoanalysis and the neurohumanities, has allowed me to reach towards an understanding of this strangest of data sets. My hope is that, in investigating this archive in such a way, I am now able to postulate that it is possible to think of the memory loss state as an alternate way of being, rather than a catastrophic loss of the self.

To try to bring a sense of an ending to something that continues to double and split and annihilate and rebuild is difficult. In the end, it is just possible to see that this archive is something that tampers with the margins of what it means to be human. It has something to do with living and dying. It has something to do with the other, and the something else. And it has something to do with the recycled parts that make up you and me. In *The Body Artist*, Don DeLillo writes, "It is about you and me. What begins in solitary otherness becomes familiar and even personal. It is about who we are when we are not rehearsing who we are."[1,2] With its uncanny ability to exist in a space which is both before and beyond the rehearsal, the read-through, and the preparation for the performance, the memory loss brain is able to show us, not only who *it* is, but who *we* are. As a lens it is simultaneously enlightening and perplexing, favouring the value of imagination and thought over the restrictions placed upon us by our human bodies that decay further with each passing chapter of time.

Learning about the memory loss experience during this study has been one of my greatest privileges. I have worked with, and learned from, participants who were living with memory loss, their carers, and their family members. I have spent time in a nursing home and observed how the nursing home environment becomes unliveable for people who are living with memory loss. I have spoken with

DOI: 10.4324/9781003639657-5

Dr Kerry Andrew and Douglas Noble about the challenges of attempting to create art that assists these diminished voices, and I have discussed the next steps in music therapy research with Dr Ming Hung Hsu. I have also had the pleasure of having two important and insightful conversations with the dementia campaigner and activist, Dr Wendy Mitchell.

Unexpected interlude

Dear Wendy,

It is the 22nd of February 2024, and I have just heard the news that you have died, which you have posthumously announced on your blog, with a post entitled, My Final Hug in a Mug; a reference to your final cup of tea.[3] *You open with, "Dear everyone who has followed my story and anyone else who cares to read this...If you're reading this, it means this has probably been posted by my daughters as I've sadly died."*[4]

You write that you had planned to end your life at the beginning of this year by visiting Dignitas in Switzerland, but a nasty fall and resultant hospital stay had meant that you had lost the confidence to fly alone, so that, in your eyes, you needed to find a way to end your own life at home. Of your method for doing so, you write, "In the end I died simply by deciding not to eat or drink any more.[SIC]"[5] *You continue with, "after my accident, the only choice open to me was to stop eating and drinking. I learnt about Voluntary Stopping Eating and Drinking (VSED) as my way out of this world during the writing of my book."*[6] *And you go on to kindly reassure your reader with, "I don't feel hunger or thirst, meaning that part of the process would be less stressful for me than for others."*[7]

I realise now that your final book, One Last Thing: How to live with the end in mind, is a thesis of sorts – a research project in which you were researching your own death.[8] *I did not read it as such when I read it, but now I am wondering how I missed it. Hearing about your death whilst I am attempting to bring this study to a close, or at least a pause, is troublesome. It at once makes perfect sense and no sense at all. You worked tirelessly during the ten years that you lived with memory loss to show how it was possible to live well with dementia, if those around us and policy makers can begin to understand what the memory loss experience feels like. You insisted that people who live with memory loss can live fulfilling lives, learn new things, enjoy a variety of creative disciplines, and have meaningful relationships with those around them. You even referred to your Alzheimer's disease as a gift.*[9] *And yet, you chose this.*

I understand why you did it; you were tired of adapting to the dementia experience, you were resolutely determined never to live in a nursing home, and you were desperate to avoid your worst fear – forgetting your daughters. Whilst I agree that your choice to accelerate your own death should have been just that; your choice, to no longer have you as a presence in this field of research feels like such an overwhelming loss. I'm sorry that ten years of masking and making sense of the changing status of your memory loss brain in a society that did not understand you left you feeling tired, and I'm sorry that you were so disappointed by the nursing home environments that you visited that ending your life prematurely felt like a more favourable option than becoming a resident in one.

You have described yourself as being optimistic, and always approaching the challenges that came with your diagnosis with a 'glass half full' approach. You write, "Dementia is a cruel disease that plays tricks on your very existence. I've always been a glass half full person, trying to turn the negatives of life around and creating positives, because that's how I cope. Well I suppose dementia was the ultimate challenge. Yes, dementia is a bummer, but oh what a life I've had playing games with this adversary of mine to try and stay one step ahead."[10] *And what a ten years you have had! Three books, two honorary doctorates, and a British Empire Medal.*[11] *You made such a difference to this field of research, and you managed to find the delicate line between acknowledging that a memory loss diagnosis is not a positive thing, whilst using education and determination to paint the memory loss experience in the most positive of lights. This is a difficult thing to do, and is a balance that I am also hoping to strike.*

My overriding concern when it comes to my work is that somebody who has had a negative experience of memory loss might read this book and think that my suggestions de-value that experience in some way. My research is about the question of value, after all, and for my words to be taken in that way would be mortifying. I hope it is clear that I am merely making suggestions for a different perspective, and I am not suggesting that anyone that thinks about the memory loss experience differently to me is incorrect.

However, what I do know is that, as a family member, thinking about the memory loss state as an alternate way of being, rather than a catastrophic loss of the self, makes it less painful, and I know this because I adopted that mindset after my grandfather was diagnosed with vascular dementia in 2017. We had the most beautiful relationship after that point and I miss him, and his brilliant memory loss brain every day.

I also know, from speaking with you, and from my fieldwork in a nursing home, that it is essential that care providers and policy makers have an understanding of the memory loss experience when working with people who are living with memory loss, so that they may make inclusive adaptations which relieve stress, promote positive wellbeing, and make the transition to and time spent in nursing homes a liveable experience. In thinking of the memory loss state as a kind of neurodiversity, and explaining that the memory loss brain is an intelligent brain, I hope I have gone some way towards making this a possibility.

Thank you, Wendy, for your time, and for giving me an insight into the wonderfully plastic nature of your memory loss brain during our two conversations. You were strong-willed, kind, funny, and ferociously intelligent. On your death, you write, "Adapting to this life with dementia is over, but I don't consider dementia has won, as that would be negative and you all know I'm a positive person. It's ME calling time on MY dementia – checkmate, before IT plays its final move."[12] *That "final move" of course being your biggest fear – forgetting your daughters. I think though, that you may have held onto that for longer than you thought, because for you, that would have been the very last thing.*

Goodbye, Wendy. I will remember you.

End of interlude

In the introduction to this book, I proposed two research questions. The first of these was, "How can a creative and critical approach to an interpretative phenomenological analysis investigation offer an insight into the memory loss experience?" My feeling is that, in using the IPA archive that I have gathered to think of the memory loss experience in terms of the uncanny, the nursing home environment, the death drive, archival impulses, prosthetic manipulation, artistic plasticity, and neuroplasticity, I have shown how the memory loss experience reacts and adapts to the loss of short-term memory, to changes to the senses, to buried trauma, and to current care practices and creative interventions. I have demonstrated how beautiful and intelligent the memory loss brain is and have shown how thinking of the memory loss state as a kind of neurodivergence opens up the possibility for a new perspective of the memory loss experience, which is inclusive, helpful, and kind. I mentioned in the second chapter of this book that the way we treat, care for, and think about people who are living with memory loss is influenced by Anne Davis Bastings, "self = memory" and "loss of memory = loss of self" and, in using the results of this study to challenge this, I am now able to suggest how this approach might begin to change, which brings me to the second of my research questions.[13]

The second research question that I proposed at the beginning of this book was, "How can data gathered during a creative and critical interpretative phenomenological analysis investigation inform suggestions for adaptations across a range of practices?" What follows are some suggestions for the way in which the findings of this research might shape future methods that aim to alleviate disorientation and help with acceptance, reducing stress and leading to better outcomes across multiple disciplines and practices, including music therapy, community musicianship, and the nursing home environment itself. These ideas have been developed entirely using the data and observations gathered during this study, and are designed to be low-cost (or, ideally, free), possible to implement without a specialist practitioner present where possible, inclusive, and accessible. All suggested interventions are also simple. This is not because I have managed to make them so using academic prowess. These interventions are simple because they *are* simple – all that they require is an openness to thinking about the memory loss experience from the perspective of which I have suggested. Please read them knowing that the suggestions come from a place of thorough research, but also of kindness and hope, even at times when they might, at first sight, appear unpalatable or disruptive.

On music

Music often had a negative impact on the participants who were living with memory loss during this study. I was not surprised by this, having observed similar reactions when performing in concerts at my late grandfather's care home. I have learned that listening to music can trigger a moment of increased lucidity, in which painful memories can be accessed, thus triggering a feeling of distress and disorientation. I have also learned that the presence of music can be challenging to people who are living with memory loss as they often choose to sit quietly or in complete silence, either as a way to 'take a break' from the sensory overload that can come with a neurodiverse state, or because they are simply enjoying a moment of calm. On this, Mitchell said,

"***Wendy:*** Sometimes just sitting in silence is the biggest help. And again in couples, there is this misunderstanding from one partner because the partner with dementia is quiet. Almost ignoring them. Well, actually, sitting in silence, this is so calming. As I said, people don't like silence. More than one thing, and it's like the wool unravelling in your head, when you have a mess instead of the calm. It's very similar to this morning when I was in selling my calendars and everybody was chatting and I couldn't focus on any conversation so I sat silently because I couldn't contribute. One woman came up to me and said, "Are you alright? You haven't said much." I explained that I can't take in all the conversations that are going on. People think there's something wrong, but you can't cope. But it's that overstimulation of stuff. It just sends you into a frazzle.

Sam: I'm really interested in what you said about listening to music, in that you find that if that's what you're doing, then that is what your brain is focused on. The listening is the task that you're doing. So I suppose if you've got music on in the background, do you find that overstimulating if you're trying to do something else?

Wendy: Yes, I don't do it. I just can't do two things at once. Even if I'm not listening to the music, it's there, and it's interrupting all the signals that my brain is giving me to do something else, because we have to concentrate so much."[14]

On a personal level, and as someone who has been a musician for 32 years, the thought that listening to music could have a negative impact on a person, whilst unsurprising due to previous observations, is something that I have found extremely challenging. I have a great love of music, and, when working as a music teacher, I have seen first-hand the positive and transformative impact that engaging with music can have. Whilst I have found that music can have a negative impact upon people who are living with memory loss, I do believe that it is possible for them to continue to enjoy and engage with music, if (a) practitioners have an understanding of the memory loss experience, and (b) if some simple adaptations are made.

On music therapy

When looking at the data collected during this study, I have several concerns about current music therapy practices for people who are living with memory loss. I wrote in the second chapter of this book that I felt as though current music therapy practices were heavily influenced by the Sacksian narrative and supported the unhelpful and exclusive "self = memory" and "loss of memory = loss of self" equation.[15] I also mentioned a conversation with Dr Ming Hung Hsu (a senior research fellow at The Cambridge Institute for Music Therapy Research with a particular interest in using music therapy with people living with memory loss) in which he explained what a 'successful' music therapy session for people who are living with memory loss might look like.[16] I wrote, "To put it simply, what happens in a conventionally successful music therapy session for a person living with memory loss is the following: a therapist plays some familiar songs in the hope that they will stimulate the brain and 'wake the person up' (as in the famous case of Henry wakes up).[17] This hopefully brings the person into a short period of lucidity, during which they are able to talk to the therapist about the memories that the song or piece of music has reminded them of."[18] This is particularly problematic in light of the data that has been gathered during this study for several reasons. I am reminded here of Participant 9's chilling second interview after she had been 'woken up' by listening to some Chopin, and also of Mitchell's comments on the problems of triggering memories from the past:

"***Wendy:*** All these reminiscence type things… you know, there were some periods in our life that we don't want to remember… Every individual has memories that they want to be recovered and memories that they don't."[19]

Here, Mitchell highlights the challenges that come with using music to trigger memories from the past, and her comments are in keeping with the reaction that Participant 9 had to listening to the piece of Chopin. My research finds, mirroring the existing canon of research, that the benefit of music therapy interventions for people who are living with memory loss is currently unclear.

In 'Music Therapy in dementia: a narrative synthesis systematic review', it was reported that, "Evidence for the benefits in music therapy in dementia remains inconclusive." and "the evidence for long-term benefits is lacking."[20,21,22] And a similar systematic review named, 'Music-based therapeutic intervention for people with dementia' found that "Providing people with dementia with at least five sessions of music-based therapeutic intervention probably reduces depressive symptoms but has little to no effect on agitation and aggression."[23,24] And it goes on to say that, "There may also be little to no effect on emotional well-being or quality of life, overall behavioural problems and cognition. We are uncertain about effects on anxiety or social behaviour and about any long-term effects."[25] My feeling is that the benefits of engaging with music therapy for people who are living with memory loss could be improved if practitioners and therapy designers had a better knowledge of the memory loss experience and made adaptations accordingly. The suggestions for adaptations to music therapy practices in Table 5.1 have been developed using my conversations with Hsu and Mitchell, my observations during my time in the nursing home, and my time spent with Participant 9.

Table 5.1 Suggestions for adaptations to music therapy practices

Suggestion for consideration	*Rationale*
In a music therapy session, therapists should **avoid the use of recognisable or 'nostalgic' pieces of music.**	Familiar music and sounds can prompt an uncanny feeling of alienation for people who are living with memory loss, which can be disorientating and unpleasant. Also, people who are living with memory loss may change their taste in music over time, so a varied range of music should be used.
When developing future music therapy designs for people who are living with memory loss, **music therapists must have a better understanding of the memory loss experience.**	Music therapists need a better understanding of the memory loss experience so that they know that, (a) accessing memories from the past can be a disorientating and upsetting experience, (b) the brief period of lucidity that listening to music induces can push people living with memory loss back into a pre-memory loss identity. This is often confusing, upsetting, and supports a negative cultural narrative that a current memory loss state has little to no value, (c) people with memory loss often spend periods of time sitting quietly. This may be because they are enjoying a moment of calm or that they are 'taking a break' from the sensory challenges that come with being in a neurodiverse state. Any attempt to 'wake them up' with music at that time is not kind, (d) there are many people who are living with memory loss who do not enjoy listening to music. The therapist should ask permission before playing music to the person. If the person is non-verbal, or unable to respond, the therapist should ask permission from a trusted individual, such as a care worker or family member who knows the person well, and (e) if playing music live, therapists should have an understanding of how to adjust their performance to make it palatable to the memory loss ear. Please see below for suggestions for adaptations to community musicianship practices.

(*Continued*)

Table 5.1 (Continued)

Suggestion for consideration	*Rationale*
Future music therapy design for people who are living with memory loss should **include 'legacy' sessions**, which are possible to achieve without the need for the presence of a music therapist.	This follows the model for current speech and language therapy practices and is vital if music therapy practices are to move beyond standalone, expensive sessions that are unaffordable for most nursing homes, thus making them inaccessible to a large proportion of people who might be living with memory loss.
A knowledge of the positive wellbeing benefits of musical learning and the memory loss brain's ability to learn new things due to neuroplasticity would be beneficial to the development of future music therapy practices for people who are living with memory loss.	People who are living with memory loss are able to keep learning new things, due to the neuroplastic nature of their brains, which is heightened due to their memory loss state. The wellbeing benefits of learning how to play or engage with musical practices are vast and should be incorporated into music therapy practices. This would stop the therapy sessions from pushing people backwards into a previous identity that they may no longer recognise and instead position them as a 'learner' in a future space in which their brain can be seen as holding value. The repetitive motor skills that come with musical learning may also serve as a useful stim which would help the person who is living with memory loss to manage the sensory challenges of their environment brought on by their neurodiverse state.

On community musicianship

Whilst I was at the nursing home, I played the flute to the residents many times. Some of these performances took place at the bedside of residents (as was the case with The Dying Artist) and some of these took place in the lounge. The performances in the lounge were generally successful, and I experimented with different ways of engaging the residents with each performance. In one session we played 'dynamics bingo', in which the residents raised their hands when the music became louder, and lowered their hands when it became quieter. On another occasion, I shared the sheet music for the music that I was playing with the residents, and they followed the music with their fingers as I played. In another session, I taught the residents some Italian musical terms (*Dolce*, meaning 'sweetly', *Cantabile*, meaning 'in a singing style', *Lento*, meaning 'slow', and *Accelerando*, meaning 'accelerating') and they listened to me play a selection of pieces and then guessed which of the terms most suited each of them. During these sessions, I learned that engaging residents in musical activities was relatively straightforward, and it was also simple to differentiate the activities to suit different needs. However, one particular resident was very difficult to engage in any musical activity, and that was Participant 4. Participant 4 (who you will remember from the second case study in chapter 3) was a pianist and found listening to and engaging with music extremely challenging, due to the changing status of her memory loss brain and ear. In her case study, I wrote, "whilst playing my fourth piece, I began to hear a familiar grumbling noise coming from Participant 4, and I wondered whether she was about to tell Participant 9 to stop crying, as she always did. The grumbling got louder and louder, and then I heard the care worker who was holding her hand say, 'You *do* like this! Don't be rude! It takes a lot of years to be able to play like that!' When I had finished playing the fourth piece, I heard that Participant 4 was in fact saying, 'It's not supposed to sound like that!' over and over again. She looked visibly distressed and refused to lift her head throughout the rest of the performance. When I had finished and was packing away, she was still repeatedly saying, 'It's not supposed to sound like that' and after that Friday morning, our relationship sadly became progressively problematic."[26] Whilst Participant 4's reaction to my performances was influenced by her personal relationship with music that had been influenced by her own musical education, her response is an example of the way in which well-meaning community musicianship practices can become negative experiences for people who are living with memory loss, if they are conducted without a knowledge of the memory loss experience. However, with some adaptations, it is possible for the performances to be positive experiences. I tested all the following suggestions for adaptations to community musicianship practices that appear in Table 5.2 during my informal performances at the nursing home. All of them were successful and made for a better, more palatable experience for the residents who were living with memory loss.

Table 5.2 Suggestions for adaptations to community musicianship practices

Adaptation	*Rationale*
Before a performance, it is necessary to **ask permission to perform.** If the person or people are non-verbal, or unable to respond, the performer may have a conversation with a trusted individual (for example, a care worker who knows the person, or a friend or family member) to ask whether they think that the person or people might enjoy/benefit from listening to some music. If the trusted person is unsure, then the performance should not take place.	Listening to music has a considerable impact upon the brain, and people should be given the choice as to whether they wish for this to happen. People living with memory loss often enjoy sitting quietly, or in silence, and a disruption to this may feel unpleasant or overwhelming. People who are living with memory loss are able to focus on one thing at a time, and they may be trying to focus on something of more value to them (a medical appointment, a visiting family member, or a different creative practice, for example) when the performance is due to take place. If this is the case then the performance should not happen.

(Continued)

Table 5.2 (Continued)

Adaptation	*Rationale*
Nostalgic programmes of music should be avoided, and performers should instead plan varied programmes that include a range of genres.	Listening to nostalgic music is particularly problematic for people who are living with memory loss, and a varied programme will cater better to the changing status of the memory loss brain, and any changes to the sense of hearing. This approach also takes into account that people who are living with memory loss may encounter a change in their taste in music.
Whilst it is possible to adapt all **instruments** for use in this context, some lend themselves more easily to the memory loss brain and ear. In general, string instruments are the most preferable, with brass, wind, and percussion, being the most problematic. However, it is possible to play instruments from these families if the performer has an awareness of the adaptations that they must make during performance. Vocalists, (particularly sopranos and descants), will also need to adhere carefully to the adaptations suggested.	When booking a community musician for a performance in a nursing home setting, instrumentation must be taken into account. If it is preferable to book a brass, wind, or percussion player, the person booking the musician should ensure that the musician is aware of the adaptations that need to be made in order to make the performance enjoyable for people who are living with memory loss.
Again, in terms of **timbre**, it is possible to play any instrument in this context, although greater care must be taken by wind, brass, and percussion players to produce a more palatable sound. In the case of wind and brass instruments, the player may choose to manage this by making a larger space within their mouths, which will create a 'woodier' sound. Imagining a rounder sound whilst performing will also help to produce this.	The warmer sound that this adaptation will create will help to make an accessible performance for people who are living with memory loss, who may have sensitive hearing, making 'harsher' sounds more difficult to listen to.
Very high **pitches** can be problematic, so minimising these is essential. For instruments that typically use higher pitches, it is recommended that performers transpose down an octave, where possible.	High pitches can be alarming and off-putting for people who are living with memory loss. This adaptation should be possible for most performers to make during the performance (with little prior planning needed) making it a simple adaptation to implement.

(*Continued*)

Table 5.2 (Continued)

Adaptation	*Rationale*
A sensitive approach to **articulation** is required. For example, a wind player should consider tonguing from the back of their mouth, rather than the front (a 'k' sound rather than a 't' sound, much like the second articulation of a double or triple tongue) in order to produce a softer articulation without losing the musical sense of the tongued note itself. Performers may also choose to use a mute, where possible.	This is one of the more nuanced ways that a performer can adapt to a memory loss audience, but it is both easy to achieve and important. Articulation need not be abandoned completely (indeed, an experienced musician would find this challenging, and it would also disrupt the overall success of the performance) but an awareness of the need for a gentler approach to articulation is another way that a performer can make a performance more enjoyable for a memory loss audience.
Vibrato should be kept to a minimum at all times, particularly in cases where a person/people are wearing a hearing aid.	A hearing aid is designed to isolate and amplify the most prominent sound. Therefore, when vibrato is used in a performance, the hearing aid will isolate only one of the undulating sounds, which will then sound like an unpleasant and intermittent alarm for a person who is wearing a hearing aid. Vibrato is often used to support intonation, so the performer should be aware of this and use other methods to ensure that a lack of vibrato means that they do not play out of tune.
At no point should the performer ask whether the person/people who are living with memory loss remember a piece of music that they have played/will play. If the performer has performed to the person/people before, **they should also avoid asking the person/people living with memory loss if they remember them.**	These questions are to be avoided as they can create a feeling of disorientation and panic for a person who is living with memory loss. If the performer is returning, a person with memory loss may not recognise them, or know why they know them, but they will remember the feeling that they had when they last met them. So, if the person enjoyed the previous performance and it made them feel happy, the sight of the performer will make them feel happy, and the opposite would be the case if the person living with memory loss had not enjoyed the performance or it had made them feel unhappy. It is likely that the person living with memory loss may not know why they feel the way that they do, or remember the previous performance, but this does not matter.

On the nursing home environment

The following suggestions for adaptations to the nursing home environment are unique to this study and have been developed using evidence from observations that I made during the time I spent in a nursing home, and the conversations that I had with Mitchell. I have mentioned previously how challenging the nursing home environment is, and I found myself to be both completely exhausted and hyper-alert from sensory overload at the end of each day that I spent there. In chapter 3, I wrote, "Upon entry, one is immediately confronted with the tinny sounds of multiple music players that work in semi-phase as they spit out strange songs of recent and recognisable pasts. These are accompanied by clinking china cups, out of tune (always flat) doorbells, earth-shaking alarms, and occasional distant and barely-there calls for help. This uncomfortable sound world is joined by a persistent wave of clashing food smells, the glare of hot, bright television screens, and the scattered ubiquitous gaze of peculiar glass eyes which watch from the worn faces of (un)familiar dolls and teddy bears."[27] This strange, unhomely home, proved to be unliveable for the residents who lived with memory loss. On this, Mitchell said;

"***Wendy:*** But in a care home, I can't get over to them how overloading for the senses it is. A lot of them think, "Oh, but we want to make it a happy place!", and you're making it the least happy place in the world if they do that. So, it's so difficult. There are very, very few people with dementia (in fact, I don't know any), that can cope with the overload, that are truly happy."[28]

And, later in the same conversation, she goes on to say;

"***Wendy:*** So, it really is about listening to people in the earliest stages, if they want to provide a really good service for those in the late stages. Otherwise the care homes are going be very empty when our generation gets to the late stage. We'll have made a home of our own! [She laughs]."[29]

Mitchell's determination not to live in a nursing home was a key factor in her decision to quicken the end of her own life using Voluntary Stopping Eating and Drinking (or, VSED) and the suggested adaptations in Table 5.3 are dedicated to her memory, with love.

Table 5.3 Suggestions for adaptations to the nursing home environment

Adaptation	*Rationale*
Turn the music off. Or, if music is playing, let that be the only thing that is happening, and encourage active listening. Active listening can happen in many ways, such as clapping the pulse, breathing in time to the pulse, talking about things people like/dislike about the music, playing dynamic 'bingo' (raising hands when the music gets louder and lowering them when it gets quieter) or encouraging people to close their eyes so that they can focus on listening to the music. Do not play the music loudly.	People who are living with memory loss are able to continue to enjoy music if it is handled sensitively, and if it is the only thing that is happening. Background music serves as an unwelcome distraction to the memory loss brain and causes a sensory overload, at which point the memory loss brain 'switches off'.
Do not try to induce a feeling of nostalgia using music or nostalgic objects.	Trying to provoke a feeling of nostalgia using music or objects can induce a forced feeling of the uncanny in people who are living with memory loss, which can be disorientating and distressing. As with my recommendations for the development of musical programmes in the field of community musicianship, it is important to note that listening to nostalgic music is particularly problematic for people who are living with memory loss, and listening to a variety of music will cater better to the changing status of the memory loss brain, and for changes to the sense of hearing. This approach also takes into account that people who are living with memory loss may encounter a change in their taste in music. The placement of nostalgic objects within the nursing home also generates an unpleasant uncanny feeling which leads to confusion and disorientation for residents who are living with memory loss. Having a range of neutral, or 'new' objects is a far less distressing practice.
Present the residents with one thing at a time. If the television is on, let that be the thing that is happening. If something else is happening, turn the television off.	People who are living with memory loss benefit from focusing on one thing at a time. When more than one thing is happening at the same time, sensory overload can occur.

(*Continued*)

Table 5.3 (Continued)

Adaptation	*Rationale*
Limit alarms, telephones, and doorbells where possible, and warn all residents before they are due to go off. Provide the residents with headphones where possible, to eliminate unwanted noise. Have a doorbell and a telephone that does not sound throughout the entire nursing home.	The environmental sound world of the nursing home environment can be distressing for people who are living with memory loss, who benefit from a calm environment, due to the neurodiverse nature of the memory loss state, but also because people who are living with memory loss are likely to have hearing aids and/or hyperacusis. These recognisable environmental sounds can also provoke a feeling of the uncanny, which may be disorientating and confusing. Limiting these sounds helps to create a space that is more liveable for a person who is living with memory loss.
If someone who is living with memory loss is sitting quietly, or even in silence, do not try to disrupt this by 'waking them up' with some entertainment.	People who are living with memory loss often enjoy sitting calmly and quietly, but it may also be a sign that they are 'taking a break' from the sensory challenges that come with being in a neurodiverse state. In either case, the kindest thing to do is not to interrupt them.

Closing thoughts

In this book, I have offered a new and valuable insight into the memory loss experience, and, in doing so, I have shown how the memory loss state might be thought of as an alternate way of being, rather than a catastrophic loss of the self. I have then used this information to design suggestions for adaptions across a variety of disciplines and practices. There is, of course, more work to be done here, but my hope is that I have demonstrated how an understanding of the experience of people who are living with memory loss opens a perspective in which the memory loss brain can hold value in a future space and can be thought of as different, not less. Finally, I must close by thanking, again, the participants of this study, for showing me how beautiful and brilliant their memory loss brains were, so that I was able to show you.

Notes

1 DeLillo, D. (2011) *The Body Artist.* London: Picador.
2 DeLillo, D. (2011) P116.
3 Mitchell, W (2024) *Which me am I today?* [online] Available at: https://whichmeamitoday.wordpress.com/blog/ [Accessed: February 22nd, 2024]

4 Mitchell, W (2024) [Accessed: February 22nd, 2024]
5 Mitchell, W (2024) [Accessed: February 22nd, 2024]
6 Mitchell, W (2024) [Accessed: February 22nd, 2024]
7 Mitchell, W (2024) [Accessed: February 22nd, 2024]
8 Mitchell, W. (2023) *One Last Thing: How to Live with the End in Mind.* London: Bloomsbury Publishing.
9 Mitchell, W. (2019) *Somebody I Used to Know.* London: Bloomsbury Publishing, p. 149.
10 Mitchell, W (2024) [Accessed: February 22nd, 2024]
11 Wharton, A. (2024) *Wendy Mitchell obituary* [online] Available at: https://www.theguardian.com/society/2024/feb/26/wendy-mitchell-obituary [Accessed: February 26th, 2024]
12 Mitchell, W (2024) [Accessed: February 22nd, 2024]
13 Davis Basting, A. (2009) *Forget Memory.* Baltimore: The John Hopkins University Press, p. 24.
14 Appendix J. www.routledge.com/9781041072652
15 Davis Basting, A. (2009) P24.
16 Appendix I. www.routledge.com/9781041072652
17 YouTube, (2022) *(Original) Man in Nursing Home Reacts to Hearing Music from his Era.* [online] Available at: https://www.youtube.com/watch?v=fyZQf0p73QM&t=43s [Accessed: May 9th, 2022]
18 See Chapter 2, PP9–28
19 Appendix CC. www.routledge.com/9781041072652
20 McDermott, O., Crellin, N., Ridder, H. M., Orrell, M. (2012) Music therapy in dementia: A narrative synthesis systematic review. *International Journal of Geriatric Psychiatry*, Volume 28, Issue 8. PP781–794. DOI: 10.1002/gps.3895
21 McDermott, O et al., (2012) P281.
22 McDermott, O et al., (2012) P281.
23 van der Steen, J. T., van Soest-Poortvliet M. C., van der Wouden, J. C., Bruinsma, M. S., Scholten, R. J., Vink, A. C. (2017) Music-based therapeutic interventions for people with dementia. *Cochrane Database of Systematic Reviews*, Issue 5. DOI: 10.1002/14651858.CD003477.pub3.
24 van der Steen, J. T. *et al.*, (2017)
25 van der Steen, J. T. *et al.*, (2017)
26 See Chapter 3, Case Study 2, Participant 4. PP45–61
27 See Chapter 3, P29.
28 Appendix CC. www.routledge.com/9781041072652
29 Appendix CC. www.routledge.com/9781041072652

Bibliography

Davis Basting, A. (2009) *Forget Memory*. Baltimore: The John Hopkins University Press.

DeLillo, D. (2011) *The Body Artist*. London: Picador.

McDermott, O., Crellin, N., Ridder, H. M., Orrell, M. (2012) Music therapy in dementia: A narrative synthesis systematic review. *International Journal of Geriatric Psychiatry*, Volume 28, Issue 8. PP781–794. DOI: 10.1002/gps.3895

Mitchell, W. (2019) *Somebody I Used to Know*. London: Bloomsbury Publishing.

Mitchell, W. (2023) *One Last Thing: How to Live with the End in Mind*. London: Bloomsbury Publishing.

Mitchell, W. (2024) *Which me am I today?* [online] Available at: https://whichmeamitoday.wordpress.com/blog/ [Accessed: March 22nd, 2024] van der Steen, J. T., van Soest-Poortvliet M. C., van der Wouden, J. C., Bruinsma, M. S., Scholten, R. J., Vink, A. C. (2017) Music-based therapeutic interventions for people with dementia. *Cochrane Database of Systematic Reviews*, Issue 5. DOI: 10.1002/14651858.CD003477.pub3.

Wharton, A. (2024) *Wendy Mitchell obituary* [online] Available at: https://www.theguardian.com/society/2024/feb/26/wendy-mitchell-obituary [Accessed: February 26th, 2024]

YouTube,(2022) *(Original) Man in Nursing Home Reacts to Hearing Music from His Era.* [online] Available at: https://www.youtube.com/watch?v=fyZQf0p73QM&t=43s [Accessed: May 9th, 2022]

Index

Note: Page references in *italics* denote figures and in **bold** tables.

FSC
www.fsc.org
MIX
Papier | Fördert
gute Waldnutzung
FSC® C083411

Kolibri 360 GmbH
Ferdinand-Jühlke-Straße 7
99095 Erfurt, Deutschland
produktsicherheit@kolibri360.de